T0203059

Borderline Personality Disorder

Brian Palmer · Brandon Unruh
Editors

Borderline Personality Disorder

A Case-Based Approach

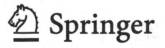 Springer

Editors
Brian Palmer
Department of Psychiatry and Psychology
Mayo Clinic
Rochester, MN
USA

Brandon Unruh
Department of Psychiatry
Harvard Medical School
McLean Hospital
Belmont, MA
USA

ISBN 978-3-319-90742-0   ISBN 978-3-319-90743-7   (eBook)
https://doi.org/10.1007/978-3-319-90743-7

Library of Congress Control Number: 2018953173

This Springer imprint is published by the registered company Springer Nature Switzerland AG
The registered company address is: Gewerbestrasse 11, 6330 Cham, Switzerland

Preface

Both of us struggled mightily on our way to becoming BPD specialists and experts. So much of the work seemed counterintuitive: making further treatment contingent on using treatment well seemed to just activate the patient's abandonment fears, then their anger, then our insecurities as young psychiatrists. Up to this point in our lives, anger was something to be accommodated and avoided – or fixed. Get curious about it? Don't take it personally? Well, not too personally…. Huh?

The early work was disorienting. What worked for other patients (and for ourselves) seemed unhelpful – even harmful – with BPD patients. Anxiety was high, sleep was disrupted, and patients were making variable progress. In the crucible of McLean Hospital's rich expertise with BPD, we found ourselves struggling to integrate and apply our training. It sometimes felt like being lost in a maze without a map, while others always knew which path to take, seated comfortably on their perches above the maze.

This book is an attempt to create that map. While it relies heavily on (and endorses principles that are generally consistent with) a number of empirically validated treatments for BPD, it is intended to be a generalist guide, a practical primer on the common and important clinical issues that routinely emerge in the treatment of people with borderline personality disorder.

We are grateful to the incredibly skilled group of contributors, all nationally recognized experts in the treatment of BPD and related conditions. They have produced chapters that balance practical guidance with nuanced discussions. We hope that the wisdom in these cases will guide clinicians in providing increasingly more effective and helpful care to patients with BPD. We are extremely grateful to John Gunderson, MD, whose influence on our thinking and patient care is amply evident on every page of this book.

The book is, of course, dedicated to our patients. While "doctor" has its roots in "teaching" and "patient" has its roots in "suffering," this is one of many examples in medicine where the words seem inverted, at least to the extent that our patients are – as has always been true in medicine – our best teachers.

Dr. Unruh would like to acknowledge that a portion of his editorial work was generously funded by donors to a McLean Borderline Personality Disorder Training Institute grant for expanding care to underserved patients.

Rochester, MN, USA   Brian Palmer, M.D., M.P.H.
Belmont, MA, USA   Brandon Unruh, M.D.

Contents

About the Editors

Brian Palmer, M.D., M.P.H. is vice chair for education and a consultant in the Department of Psychiatry and Psychology at Mayo Clinic. Following graduation from Mayo Clinic School of Medicine, he served as national president of the American Medical Student Association before completing his psychiatry residency at MGH/McLean in Boston. He joined the staff of McLean Hospital, specializing in borderline personality disorder (BPD) and working closely with John Gunderson, MD, with whom he continues to teach several times yearly. At Mayo Clinic, he oversees the department's educational mission, including continuing education, patient education, the medical student clerkship, and the department education committee. He is medical director of the Transitions Program, an outpatient day treatment program, serving primarily patients with BPD. His research interests are in personality disorders and their interface with mood disorders.

Brandon Unruh, M.D. is an instructor in psychiatry at Harvard Medical School and a specialist in personality disorders at McLean Hospital in Belmont, Massachusetts. He is a graduate of Harvard University and the UCLA School of Medicine, and he completed psychiatry residency training at Massachusetts General and McLean Hospital. He came to a career in psychiatry and psychotherapy – and eventually personality disorders – through interests in the broad questions posed by literature, religion, and philosophy. His clinical work, academic interests, and teaching are anchored in the integration of evidence-based treatments for personality disorders such as mentalization-based treatment, dialectical behavioral therapy, transference-focused psychotherapy, and good psychiatric management. He is the director of the Mentalization-Based Treatment (MBT) Training Clinic, assistant director of the Borderline Personality Disorder Training Institute, and assistant medical director of the Gunderson Residence at McLean Hospital. He teaches and supervises psychiatry residents and other trainees and published the first standardized residency curriculum for BPD.

Contributors

Steven Bartek, M.D. Department of Psychiatry, University of Michigan, Ann Arbor, MI, USA

Claire Brickell, M.D. McLean Hospital and Harvard Medical School, Belmont, MA, USA

Stephanie H. Cho, M.D. Department of Psychiatry and Behavioral Sciences, Keck School of Medicine of the University of Southern California, Los Angeles, CA, USA

Robert P. Drozek, LICSW McLean Hospital, Belmont, MA, USA

Carl Fleisher, M.D. UCLA, Department of Psychiatry and Biobehavioral Sciences, Los Angeles, CA, USA

Victor Hong, M.D. Department of Psychiatry, University of Michigan, Ann Arbor, MI, USA

Karen Jacob, Ph.D. Gunderson Residence, McLean Hospital, Belmont, MA, USA

Department of Psychiatry, Harvard Medical School, Cambridge, MA, USA

James A. Jenkins, M.D. Harvard Medical School, McLean Hospital, Belmont, MA, USA

Carlene MacMillan, M.D. Brooklyn Minds, Psychiatry, P.C. and Ellenhorn, L.L.C., New York, NY, USA

Sara Rose Masland, Ph.D. Department of Psychology, Pomona College, Claremont, CA, USA

Benjamin McCommon, M.D. Department of Psychiatry, Columbia University, New York, NY, USA

Owen Muir, M.D. Brooklyn Minds, Brooklyn, NY, USA

Brian Palmer, M.D., M.P.H. Mayo Clinic, Department of Psychiatry and Psychology, Rochester, MN, USA

Daniel Price, M.D. Department of Psychiatry, Maine Medical Center, Tufts University School of Medicine, Portland, ME, USA

Elsa Ronningstam, Ph.D. Harvard Medical School, Department of Psychiatry, McLean Hospital, Belmont, MA, USA

Zeina Saliba, M.D. Department of Psychiatry & Behavioral Sciences, George Washington University, Washington, DC, USA

Department of Obstetrics & Gynecology, Virginia Commonwealth University, Richmond, VA, USA

Maureen Smith, LICSW McLean Hospital, Belmont, MA, USA

Brandon Unruh, M.D. McLean Hospital, Harvard Medical School, Belmont, MA, USA

Igor Weinberg, Ph.D. McLean Hospital/Harvard Medical School, Belmont, MA, USA

Joan Wheelis, M.D. Department of Psychiatry, Harvard Medical School, McLean Hospital, Belmont, MA, USA

Organizing and Shaping a Treatment Toward Change

Brian Palmer and Brandon Unruh

Case Introduction

Isabel is a 21-year-old woman who established care with you several months ago after a chaotic series of repeated overdoses, dropping out of college, multiple hospitalizations, and a family that was at the breaking point – mom sleeping outside her door in hopes of preventing another suicide attempt, and dad threatening to hire 24-h security to keep her safe. Treatment began reasonably well. You referred the parents to a Family Connections group that provided psycho-education about BPD and taught them skills for responding effectively to Isabel and managing their own distress about her problems. They described the group as a "godsend" and grew less anxious and more understanding of Isabel. Her autobiography was a useful entrée into her inner life; she has always struggled with her adoption and unwanted sexual experiences with a neighborhood boy of her age when she was 8 and 9. She felt understood by you, her urges to die decreased, she stopped bingeing/purging, and the family expressed gratitude for your care. You have repeatedly suggested (for 6 weeks in a row) that she get a part-time job, and she agrees in session but takes no steps toward applying for work between sessions.

B. Palmer, M.D., M.P.H. (✉)
Mayo Clinic, Department of Psychiatry and Psychology, Rochester, MN, USA

B. Unruh, M.D.
McLean Hospital, Harvard Medical School, Belmont, MA, USA

© Springer International Publishing AG, part of Springer Nature 2018
B. Palmer, B. Unruh (eds.), *Borderline Personality Disorder*,
https://doi.org/10.1007/978-3-319-90743-7_1

Choice Point 1

For each choice point, choose H: "helpful," U: "unhelpful or harmful," or P: "perhaps helpful, with reservations".

With regard to Isabel's lack of progress on the job front, would you:

1. Continue to provide gentle encouragement each week (keep the status quo)
2. Make further work with you contingent on part-time (or full-time) work, a regular volunteer position, or part-time school.
3. Bring in her parents to emphasize the importance of work and enlist their support.
4. Wonder if her avoidance of work is an attempt to insure that her parents will care for and protect her, linking to how she may have felt they failed to protect her as a child.
5. Let the job issue go for now because work may increase her symptoms and she may be wise to keep things manageable.

Discussion

At this point, the treatment is off to a good start. Symptoms have been reduced, likely through stabilizing the home environment and experiencing you as a trusted other. But the case is at a precarious point. In addition to useful relationship with you, the other factor related to symptom improvement is the avoidance of interpersonal stressors that were likely present at school and would be present on a job. Further avoidance poses real risks for both this young woman's life trajectory and a treatment that could easily become unhelpful. If you give up on the job push (or simply continue to try your gentle encouragement for several more weeks), then Isabel is unlikely to move forward in life outside of treatment. Being clear that work or school is part of her treatment is entirely consistent with good care – it anchors the treatment in an expectation of functional improvement.

Data from both the McLean Study of Adult Development (MSAD) [1, 2] and the Collaborative Longitudinal Personality Disorders Study (CLPS) [3] show convincingly that BPD symptoms improve. Eighty percent of patients no longer meet diagnostic criteria in 10 years, and once remission of symptoms is achieved, relapse is rare. However, both of these studies show that functional improvement is limited. In CLPS, only a third of the sample had a stable job at the end of 10 years.

Enlisting the parents to shape the patient's behavior has problems for both roles and goals. At the same time, if the parents were to be "enlisted," it could be helpful if done in specific manner. A common mistake that parents make is decreasing support when a patient is moving forward (college, job, etc.) and increasing support during crises. It may be useful to advise the parents (in front of the patient) that you believe that getting a job will be a real challenge and will require their emotional support for her efforts in moving forward.

Regarding the interpretation in choice 4, there may (or may not) be a morsel of truth in the question, but pursuing that approach would likely serve to justify her avoidance of work rather than help her approach the issue directly.

It is probable that her symptoms may increase when beginning a job. Expecting this and anticipating the difficulties can be very helpful.

Answers

1. U
2. H
3. P
4. U
5. U

Principles and Clinical Pearls

1. Anchoring the treatment in life outside of the therapy helps insure that the treatment has benefit for the patient's life, social roles, and functioning.
2. Complicity with a patient's avoidance of work or school can contribute to regressive treatments that improve symptoms primarily through avoidance.
3. Anticipating with a patient and family that a new job or return to school would be expected to cause a transient increase in symptoms (and therefore benefit from increased support) can help set up success.

Case Continues...

You again bring up the job issue and tell her directly that further work with you is contingent on her establishing part-time (or full-time) work, a regular volunteer position, or part-time school in the next 4 weeks. She bursts into tears and yells that she knew you would just want to "kick me to the curb" if you knew any real details of her life.

Choice Point 2

With regard to Isabel's protest that you do not care, how would you respond?

1. "I'm rooting for you to succeed because I believe you're special."
2. "Criticizing me isn't likely to help you get a job."
3. "That's a painful thought. My insistence on the job is, at least in my mind, because I want to help you."
4. "Tell me more about your feeling that I don't care."

Discussion

One of the challenges that clinicians face comes in interventions that they know will activate the patient's symptoms and especially their anger (see "Clinician Experience" sidebar). In this case, encouraging work is a key to the case, and the decision to make further treatment contingent on progress in this regard is good practice. Nonetheless, this then activates the patient.

The "sweet spot" is in both acknowledging the patient's experience and holding the position that a job is necessary. Choice 3 does this in two ways, including labeling the patient's thought as a thought and clarifying motivation, while holding firm on the contingency.

Choice 1 overcompensates and may function to undo the clinician's own feelings of guilt by reverting back to a supportive stance or creating a sense of special relationship. Choice 2 is factually true but unhelpfully sarcastic and fails to acknowledge the clinician's presence as a person in the relationship. The irreverence, though, could have a place in an established relationship like this one if it is consistent with the clinician's usual style. Choice 4 is unnecessarily explorative and contains neutrality that is disingenuous. At the same time, the anger at you is an important phenomenon that likely relates to the patient's desire for noncontingent support and activation of her symptoms in the setting of feeling challenged (and equating/relating the challenge with a sense of her own badness). It is a topic worthy of discussion.

Answers

1. U
2. U
3. H
4. P

Principles and Clinical Pearls

1. Anchoring treatment in observable life improvements can elicit fears of criticism and abandonment; addressing these directly in the context of treatment goals can help.

Case Continues...

She returns the next week and tells you that she has applied for several part-time jobs and interviewed yesterday at a local animal shelter and has been offered a job. She states that her parents were very pleased to hear this. She tells you that she has always loved animals and acknowledges that she is looking forward to the chance to care for the animals at the shelter.

Choice Point 3

How would you respond to Isabel's news about her job?

1. "Congratulations! I am glad you followed through and am happy for you."
2. "Have you considered that some of these animals will be put down?"
3. "Nice work – glad you were able to get an interview, and this sounds like a good fit for your interests. What challenges do you anticipate?"
4. "What is it like to have your mother pleased with you?"
5. "How did you prepare for that interview, and what do you think helped it go so well?"

Discussion

An important BPD clinical pearl is that progress evokes fears of abandonment. In this case, the challenge is to balance complimenting the patient while supporting how hard this progress is and how she will need more, not less, support with this success. Choice 3 attempts to demonstrate this balance, whereas choice 1 errs on the complimentary slide, and choice 2 errs on the side of holding out the difficulty without acknowledging the step forward.

Choice 4 is a potentially interesting question in this case, but it moves into an intrapsychic realm at a moment that the patient is focused on moving forward into her life. Choice 5 demonstrates a useful approach that takes a different tack: scrutinizing the success. In this approach, the success is acknowledged in a way that helps the patient consider what she did to achieve it. This helps avoid being too rosy about the achievement and refocuses the session on the role that the patient had in the achievement. If used, combining with some aspect of number 3 would be ideal.

Answers

1. U
2. U
3. H
4. U
5. H

Principles and Clinical Pearls

1. Scrutinizing successes can help patients to consider their own role in creating the success.
2. Progress evokes abandonment fears; predicting struggles during transitions helps with success.

Case Continues...

As you and she predicted, she did have an increase in symptoms in her first two weeks at the new job. She was fearful that she would make a mistake (forgetting to feed an animal was the worst mistake she imagined) and hurt or kill one of the animals under her care. You asked a bit more about that, and she volunteered that she may be catastrophizing just a bit; you both laughed. She was able to talk more about a fear of a more likely event: that she would become overly concerned with an animal not being adopted and have difficulty tolerating the animal's loneliness. You wondered if maybe her own sensitivity to aloneness was part of this picture; "yeah, I can see how that might be relevant." At this point, you believe the treatment is progressing well both inside and outside of the room with you.

Then... the patient returns the next week to share that she has a new boyfriend. She had been spending time on several online dating sites over the last few weeks, unbeknownst to you. She shared that she had a few dates with various guys and thinks she finally found "the one" in Justin, whom she has now met three times. Justin is a 42-year-old man who has been married twice before and who works part time. She is most excited about the fact he rides a motorcycle, and she feels "very safe" when she is with him.

Choice Point 4

How would you respond to Isabel's announcement about her newfound relationship?

1. Offer a supportive comment about being happy for her moving forward in a relationship.
2. Inquire about what she means when she describes "feeling safe" and provide education about BPD and being preoccupied with connecting in a relationship.
3. Tell her that you predict this relationship will not go well.

This question attempts to elucidate the therapeutic frame of helping the patient make sense of her inner experiences (in this case, helping her sees her longing and behavior with greater perspective), offering practical life guidance, and anticipating problems together with the patient. Choice 1 is unnecessarily neutral – there are obvious problems that Isabel is about to run into, and this is an opportunity to help increase her awareness of her experience and think more carefully about her decisions. Choice 2 effectively meets the needs of the moment. Choice 3 misses the opportunity to help the patient who considers her own experience in favor of you telling her about her experience; expressing your concern is certainly reasonable, but expressing it in a way that is closer to her experience will be more helpful.

Answers

1. U
2. H
3. P

Principles and Clinical Pearls

1. When present, linking behaviors to BPD's interpersonal hypersensitivity can help make the patient's experience more explicit.

Case Continues...

She elects to tell her parents about Justin and brings him to the house. Her father (who is a year older than Justin) becomes enraged and tells Justin that he is never to see Isabel again. Isabel, screaming and in tears, runs from the house to leave with Justin on his motorcycle. Her mother calls you, desperate, and you express concern and agree with her plan to text her daughter (who does respond to her mother that she is safe but upset). You encourage the parents to decrease their own reactivity and remind them that their daughter has a disorder that includes impulsive decision making, intolerance of aloneness, and chaotic relationships; their job is to be stable, predictable, and reliable. You further encourage mom to text a supportive note that Isabel is welcome home when she wants to come back. Isabel returns home after 2 days and tells her mother that Justin quickly determined that he was not interested in a relationship and agreed to drop her off at a friend's house. She has eaten very little and did not go to work (resulting in termination from this new job). She went to her room at and threw a framed picture of her and her father against the wall, shattering the glass, which she then used to superficially scratch her left forearm. Her mother alerts you to the situation, and you ask to speak with Isabel, who, crying, tells you she has lost everything and everyone and asks if you can help. You ascertain that the wound does not need medical attention and tell her you had like to see her at your standing appointment the next day.

Choice Point 5

At your next session, what will be most important?

1. Examine how she became symptomatic again, assuming that it had to do with gaining and losing external support.
2. Recommend an Intensive Outpatient Program or higher level of care, given the severity of her recent behavior.

3. Make a plan for her day structure and review her crisis plan.
4. Ask if she is having thoughts of suicide, and if so, plan to hospitalize her.
5. Tell her that further work with you is contingent on no further cutting.

Discussion

At least two goals should dominate the session. First, this series of events begs for a chance to understand what has gone on, particularly as it relates to support and the perception of losing support. At the same time, there is a need to address the new lack of day structure (which will likely contribute to worsening symptoms) and re-address safety planning and a skillful approach to managing crises. Secondarily, the parents will likely feel free to be more supportive if a written crisis plan can be shared with them. Reminding everyone that Isabel has a role in managing her safety, and behavior should help the parents who avoid the urge to grow more controlling in the face of recent events.

Choices 1 and 3 together reflect the needed approach. Regarding level of care that assessment is certainly going to be a part of the session, but at this point, the patient has demonstrated her ability to keep her appointment with you and is engaged in outpatient treatment, so the bias would be toward keeping her as an outpatient. That said, an IOP could help with skill building and day structure while she applies for a new job, and if she was interested it could certainly be helpful. If she has increased internal agitation and hopelessness on your observation of her mental status during your session or if she has continued to be impulsive and destructive, an IOP may be a very good option. Hospitalization should be reserved for an acute suicidal crisis. Certainly if she feels unloveable and has a tunnel vision toward suicide in your session, hospitalization may be important for her safety. But superficial scratching in the setting of an interpersonal crisis should not, in and of itself, trigger a move toward hospitalization, which – based on the data provided – would likely do more harm than good. Bringing up termination at this point is unwise; the behavioral episode is worth understanding and addressing, but the treatment at this point remains on track.

Answers

1. H
2. P
3. H
4. U
5. U

Principles and Pearls

1. When a patient is activated (angry, anxious, self-injurious), increasing external structure and support can be stabilizing and allow for reflection and planning around stressors that are likely to recur.

Summary of Clinical Approach

This case captures several key principles of working with a patient with BPD. The first is to consider the interpersonal context for the symptoms. Symptoms reduce with increased support (though this can lead to regressive treatments), and they increase with transitions and interpersonal stressors. Grounding a treatment in the expectation of functional progress is a key principle, given the troubling data that most patients with BPD improve symptomatically but not functionally. Moreover, such an approach also helps steer clear of complicity with avoidance-based symptom improvement. Families are a key to treatment. They have many of the same concerns and reactions as treaters do, and helping them to learn skills to decrease their own reactivity can be extremely helpful. The case also emphasizes practical, here-and-now approaches which are not incompatible with deeper interpretations but which are accessible and help anchor and stabilize the work.

Clinician Experience: Aversion to Anger

A common barrier to effective management of BPD is discomfort with anger, either within oneself or the patient. Many clinicians shrink back from insisting on functional progress in work or school as a condition of ongoing treatment to avoid angering or alienating patients who feels their difficulties with moving forward in life is unappreciated. The "path of least resistance" for clinicians is to continue indefinitely seeing patients who value a supportive therapeutic relationship but fearfully avoid orienting themselves around real-world demands that present the possibility of failure. Clinicians may hope that through longer term alliance building the patient may eventually come around to seeing the wisdom of the recommendation to work. However, this approach fails to appreciate how tightly BPD patients cling to relationships that support their avoidance of making changes that are needed but terrifying.

What works best is to "put some teeth" into practical recommendations by making treatment contingent on demonstrating progress. This requires anticipating, feeling comfortable with, and "leaning into" patients' predictably angry responses to such an approach. Activating anger within a therapeutic relationship by underscoring the need to change is far preferred to mutual avoidance of this reality. Once anger is openly expressed in the face of pressure to change, it helps to tell patients that you welcome the direct expression of anger and also empathize with its source in their fears of failure. Both interventions preserve a sense of connection and help restabilize the therapeutic relationship over time following acutely angry responses jarring to both patient and clinician.

Especially early on in learning to work with BPD patients, this stance runs counter to many clinicians' temperament and default stance. In our experience, if the difficulty stems from the clinician's own discomfort with anger, it can be improved and shaped over time through educating oneself about the key role of anger in BPD phenomenology, supervision, personal psychotherapy to resolve one's own conflicts around handling anger, and collaboration with senior clinicians who can model the effectiveness of dealing with anger head-on.

References

1. Zanarini MC, Frankenburg FR, Reich DB, Fitzmaurice G. Time to attainment of recovery from borderline personality disorder and stability of recovery: a 10-year prospective follow-up study. Am J Psychiatry. 2010;167(6):663–7.
2. Zanarini MC, Frankenburg FR, Reich DB, Fitzmaurice G. The 10-year course of psychosocial functioning among patients with borderline personality disorder and axis II comparison subjects. Acta Psychiatr Scand. 2010;122(2):103–9.
3. Gunderson JG, Stout RL, et al. Ten-year course of borderline personality disorder: psychopathology and function from the collaborative longitudinal personality disorders study. Arch Gen Psychiatry. 2011;68(8):827–37.

Stimulating Reflection and Curiosity

Robert P. Drozek

Choice Point Index
1. Utilizing empathic validation as a primary intervention to address black-and-white thinking in BPD
2. Exploring how patients arrive at their more black-and-white perspectives
3. Sharing one's own viewpoint to stimulate further reflection and curiosity
4. Attempting surprising and unexpected interventions when patients are disconnected from their thoughts and feelings
5. Exploring the deeper meaning of patients' concrete demands
6. Empathically validating patients' emotions and transparently sharing one's own perspective about patients' demands

Case Introduction

Luke is a 25-year-old man referred to you initially for treatment of depression. A graduate student in English literature, he has been struggling with social isolation, poor motivation, and feelings of worthlessness. While he self-identifies as gay, he has never had a romantic interaction with a man, and he describes intense feelings of shame about his sexual orientation. As you get to know Luke better, you observe many symptoms consistent with borderline personality disorder (BPD): an unstable sense of self-esteem, intense and highly changeable emotional states, powerful feelings of emptiness, suicidal fantasies, and self-injurious behaviors such as scratching and occasional cutting. These symptoms arise in the context of Luke's interpersonal challenges – comparing himself negatively with other students in his graduate program, feeling criticized by his parents, and

R. P. Drozek, LICSW
McLean Hospital, Belmont, MA, USA
e-mail: rdrozek@mclean.harvard.edu

© Springer International Publishing AG, part of Springer Nature 2018
B. Palmer, B. Unruh (eds.), *Borderline Personality Disorder*,
https://doi.org/10.1007/978-3-319-90743-7_2

being alone for extended periods of time, during which he feels like "a loser" who is fundamentally incapable of relationships.

You review the BPD diagnosis with Luke, providing education about its etiology, course, and effective treatment. He responds enthusiastically, sharing that it explains and validates the range of difficulties with which he has struggled for most of his life. He becomes a "star student" of BPD – purchasing and devouring books about the diagnosis, joining online message boards, and journaling dutifully about his moment-to-moment emotional fluctuations. He becomes attached to you as a therapist, and he reports improvements in his mood and level of motivation.

Several weeks into the therapy, Luke arrives appearing on-edge, serious, and despondent. Through gritted teeth, he explains slowly and quietly that he attended a family dinner with his parents and siblings over the weekend. His siblings shared extensively about their professional successes and family relationships, and Luke increasingly began to feel like "a horrible loser," concluding that his hard work in therapy will never help him get better or lead a "normal life" like his siblings.

Choice Point 1

For each intervention, choose H: "helpful," U: "unhelpful or harmful," or P: "perhaps helpful, with reservations."

You consider making the following comments to Luke:

1. "You seem to be struggling with some very intense emotions right now. Could we review some distress tolerance skills together, to help you calm down?"
2. "Could you explain further what makes you feel like such a loser?"
3. "Are you able to consider some of your positive attributes, or any other evidence against this idea that you're a loser?"
4. "This sounds like a horrible experience – you feel like a complete loser, and it's difficult for you to imagine that changing in any way."

Discussion

One of the most vexing challenges of working with patients with BPD is addressing their tendencies toward extreme and rigid forms of experiencing, commonly described as "black-and-white thinking." Patients in this mode seem unreflectively certain of their perspectives, often using absolute and non-nuanced language like "always" and "never," "everyone" and "no one," "perfect" and "evil." One way that therapists can help in such moments is to stimulate greater reflection and curiosity. This increased flexibility of mind renders patients less vulnerable to core BPD-related problems such as interpersonal instability, emotional dysregulation, and self-injury.

In the current session, you have noted the black-and-white quality of Luke's thinking. All listed potential interventions seem geared toward generating increased flexibility about his conception of himself as a hopeless "loser," but some are more likely to work than others. Option 3 risks intensifying Luke's rigid attachment to his perspective by leading him to feel his current intense emotional experience is unappreciated by you, and to "dig in his heels" by further insisting on the hopelessness of his situation.

In contrast, Option 4 constitutes a basic form of *empathic validation*, a technical approach common to most evidence-based treatments for BPD [4]. Perhaps paradoxically, it is often most helpful to articulate and empathize with the patient's current affective experience before attempting to stimulate greater reflection upon it. As Luke feels better understood by you, he is likely to feel less overwhelmed, work less at getting you to see his hopelessness, and become receptive to more challenging or change-oriented interventions.

While asking Luke to clarify and elaborate his reasons for self-negativity might prove useful (Option 2), he is likely to do this in a more meaningful and curious way once you have first validated his current intense experience.

Furthermore, although skills are generally helpful for patients with BPD and there might be some value in temporarily shifting Luke's focus away from emotionally charged experiences, skills-based interventions at this moment (Option 1) could sidestep an opportunity to help Luke increase his curiosity about his negative self-conception.

Answers

1. U
2. P
3. U
4. H

Principles and Clinical Pearls

1. The ability to reflect meaningfully on one's own experiences is inversely related to the intensity of one's emotional arousal. Empathic validation is a foundational intervention that can help patients with BPD feel well-enough understood to begin reconsidering their unreflective "all-or-nothing" perspectives.

Case Continues...

You decide to respond to Luke emphatically: "This sounds like a horrible experience—you feel like a complete loser, and it's difficult for you to imagine that changing in any way." Luke appears genuinely taken aback, stammering back to you in a normal tone of voice, "Yes… that's exactly what I feel."

Choice Point 2

How do you respond to Luke in this moment?

1. Invite Luke to share more about his childhood relationships with his parents, to encourage reflection about the developmental precursors to his low self-esteem.
2. Ask Luke to discuss his reasons for seeing himself in this way: "How do you arrive at this sense of yourself?"
3. Highlight the positive attributes Luke's negative self-concept appears to ignore: his academic successes, positive relationships with his family, diligence, and intelligence.

Discussion

Your empathic validation appears to have taken Luke by surprise, helped him feel calmer, and shifted his focus away from proving his worthlessness to you. He is now likely more receptive to reflecting further about the sources, scope, and impact of this experience.

Asking Luke to reflect on his childhood relationships (Option 1) risks focusing his attention on a topical area that seems meaningful to you, but may not be to him. Because he values his relationship with you, he might be led to prematurely agree with your ideas rather than deploy his own reflectiveness to identify thoughts and experiences meaningful to him for joint exploration. In this way, BPD treatments can often appear meaningful to therapists and yet remain unimpactful for patients.

Drawing Luke's attention to his successes (Option 3) could be perceived as a subtle way of "arguing with" his inflexible viewpoint, generating a power struggle that might shut down his reflectiveness. Alternatively, were he to embrace a positive sense of himself merely on the strength of your suggestion, this approach risks Luke becoming overly reliant on *your* views about him, rather than reconsidering his own.

By inviting Luke to elaborate on his reasons for seeing himself so negatively (Option 2), you would be helping him to develop a more reflective and nuanced perspective on that negativity. Asking him to explain and explore his justification for a viewpoint implies that we are focusing on *a viewpoint*, rather than a veridical representation of reality. Furthermore, because this intervention does not seek to contradict Luke's negative self-concept, it could provide further empathic resonance with how strongly he is attached to it. This lays important emotional groundwork for further reflection and curiosity about his position over time.

Answers

1. U
2. H
3. U

Principles and Clinical Pearls

1. Once the therapist has validated the patient's rigidly held perspectives, asking questions like "How did you reach that conclusion?" and "What makes you see things this way?" offers an opportunity to develop higher level of reflection and curiosity about the perspective in question.

Case Continues...

You decide to ask Luke further about what makes him see himself as such a hopeless "loser." He elaborates a host of self-judgments about his lack of meaningful friendships, his unrequited romantic interests, and his failure to achieve a successful career like his siblings. As he discusses these matters, his tone becomes lighter and more conversational, and the expression on his face begins to soften. He concludes by saying that it is hard for him to imagine ever having a romantic relationship.

Choice Point 3

You consider making the following comments to Luke:

1. "You said 'hard' to imagine ever having a romantic relationship, not 'impossible' to imagine. What were you getting at there?"
2. "You just feel so horrible about yourself, like such a loser who will never get better."
3. "As I hear you list these self-criticisms, I am finding myself wanting to highlight some of your *positive* traits, some of the good things about you."
4. "You are discussing so many things that have not happened in your life yet, but it does not follow that they *will never* happen. You are just starting therapy, which will hopefully help you with these matters."

Discussion

Luke now appears to have moved into a stance of greater reflection about his experiences. Option 1 highlights the softening of Luke's language and his possible shift toward a less black-and-white perspective about his future. Doing so implicitly encourages and reinforces his deepening reflective process. Option 3 aims to spur reflection along a different channel, by sharing your own (more positive) perspective without attempting to change Luke's own perspective. This invites him to consider the discrepancy between your two perspectives, which could lead to a higher level of curiosity about why he clings so tightly to his own. One disadvantage of sharing your mind so transparently is that it misses an opportunity to extend the reflective moves Luke is already making of his own accord.

On the other hand, prolonged attempts at empathic validation (Option 2) risk amplifying Luke's hopelessness by overly joining with a viewpoint he was just beginning to question. Option 4 explicitly challenges Luke's pessimism by drawing upon your own optimism and reflective process, rather than attending to how these processes are unfolding for him.

Answers

1. H
2. U
3. P
4. U

Principles and Clinical Pearls

1. As patients move into positions of increased reflection and curiosity about their experiences, the therapist should "stop the presses" to explicitly observe these productive shifts, and encourage and validate the reflective processes that are unfolding.

Case Continues...

You observe that Luke mentioned that it was "hard" but not "impossible" for him to imagine having a romantic relationship. He confirms that he often feels like he will *never* have a romantic relationship with someone, but sometimes is more optimistic.

As therapy continues over the next several months, Luke reports improvements in his self-confidence, self-esteem, and hope for the future. He continues to struggle with nagging fears that he will never get better but feels less certain that these transient experiences confirm a dismal future. His self-injury begins to decrease.

Luke arrives for today's session appearing anxious, distracted, and on-edge, reporting that he is "depressed." When asked to elaborate, he responds, "I'm just depressed... it's just how I always am – there's nothing more to say about it."

Choice Point 4

You consider responding to Luke in the following ways:

1. "I hear you saying you're depressed, but from where I am sitting, you seem a bit anxious and on-edge."
2. "Of course you're feeling depressed. How about we review some coping strategies that might help you feel better?"

3. "Well, 'depression' means different things to different people. Could you try to say a little bit more about what *your* depression feels like?"
4. "Can you tell me a bit about what's been happening in your life lately?"

Discussion

In an earlier session, Luke was rigidly nonreflective about his experience. In the current session, it is not clear if Luke is even *connected* with his experience – he is using the word "depressed" but does not objectively appear depressed. When attempting to stimulate curiosity in such moments, the primary therapeutic task is to do whatever you can to help patients start to authentically access their own experiences. We cannot reflect on an experience (e.g., a thought, emotion, or desire) from which we are disconnected.

Reviewing depression-related coping strategies (Option 2) is unlikely to help, as it would assume Luke is accurately and meaningfully describing his emotions. Asking about Luke's idiosyncratic experience of "depression" (Option 3) is more promising, because it sidesteps the trappings of undescriptive labels and refocus attention to his interior *experience*. However, this approach risks inviting potentially unproductive further discourse about himself as merely "depressed," which seems to be an unreflective signifier of more a multifaceted experience.

In contrast, Options 1 and 4 more fully circumvent Luke's focus on the word "depression." Drawing attention to Luke's anxious appearance (Option 1) directs his attention to the here-and-now and to your own impression of his emotional state. This might prompt a more meaningful consideration of his current emotional experience. Inquiring about Luke's recent life events (Option 4) could engender reflection and genuineness by surprising him and "changing the subject" to a different area that is still meaningfully related to his presenting complaint.

Answers

1. H
2. U
3. P
4. H

Principles and Clinical Pearls

1. When patients appear to be disconnected from their experiences, the primary therapeutic task is to help them access and represent those experiences in a meaningful way.
2. In such moments, it is usually most helpful to fundamentally "shift the frame" of therapeutic discourse, either by directing their attention to here-and-now events

within the clinical interaction, or to attempt more surprising interventions that might jolt them into a position of more meaningful reflection.

Case Continues...

You decide to share your impression of Luke as being quite anxious and on-edge. He responds, "Well, I guess I am quite anxious, but really the depression is what is most painful to me right now." You invite him to say more about what has been upsetting him so much, and he reveals that he recently met a man on an online dating site. Through increasing online communication, Luke imagines they have built a genuine connection. These developments have been exciting but also distressing, given his shame about his sexuality and his fears about starting a romantic relationship. A first date is planned.

You next see Luke immediately following the date. He enters sobbing, saying that his online interest did not show, and he was left waiting alone in a coffee shop. He describes this as his ultimate fear of being rejected just after allowing himself to get close to another person. You empathize with his feelings of abandonment and name this as an important focus for your session today. Luke looks up and, with a serious expression on his face, tells you that what he really needs today is for you to give him a hug. He wants "to be held and told that everything will be okay."

Choice Point 5

In this moment, you consider employing the following interventions:

1. Give Luke a hug but keep it brief and tell him this is a one-time occurrence.
2. Ignore Luke's request and gently inquire about the circumstances of the date.
3. Inform Luke that the ethical guidelines of your profession prohibit you from hugging him, but you remain dedicated to helping him in other ways.
4. Ask Luke to share further about how a hug from you would be helpful.

Discussion

Luke's request exemplifies another particularly challenging feature of working with patients with BPD – their tendency to overly focus on external, directly observable factors as infallible indicators of internal states of mind. In this experiential mode, the only way patients can feel "okay" is if something concrete happens in their environment. This mode of being can lead to many of the characteristically "impulsive" patterns of these patients, including suicidal thinking and gestures, risk-taking behaviors, and rage and demandingness in their relationships with others. Clinicians working with patients in this frame of mind often experience powerful impulses to "meet action with action," for example by complying with patients' demands against better clinical judgment. The primary therapeutic task in such moments is to provoke higher level reflection about the needs being expressed and the demands being made. Doing so helps patients develop increased impulse control.

Accordingly, hugging Luke (Option 1) would convey that you fully share his assumption that he "needs" a hug and cannot solve his problem otherwise. In addition to violating ethical codes of professional conduct, this response fails to encourage reflection about his current needs and their form of expression. Although ignoring Luke's request (Option 2) more appropriately maintains boundaries, it emphasizes a different form of action (*your* avoidance of discussing the "elephant in the room") rather than cultivating shared reflection and curiosity about his request. Avoiding addressing an uncomfortable request may momentarily ease your nerves, but it problematically colludes with Luke's experience of his impulse as overwhelming and overpowering.

The most helpful approach involves inquiring further about Luke's desire for a hug from you (Option 4). You do not yet fully understand what his request means to him, and Luke would also benefit from considering more carefully what has driven him to make it. Stating directly that you will not hug Luke (Option 3) might be necessary at some point, but doing so *before* asking him to elaborate on his wish might communicate criticism and rejection, which in turn could inhibit higher reflection.

Answers

1. U
2. U
3. P
4. H

Principles and Clinical Pearls

1. When patients request or demand concrete responses from clinicians, there can be a powerful impulse to "do something" in response. Withholding action in such moments allows for a more productive exploration of the emotional meaning of patients' requests while modeling a reflective form of impulse control.

Case Continues...

You ask Luke to share further about how he imagines a hug from you would be helpful. He explains that, through your work together, he has become increasingly able to access his desires for closeness with others. In his mind, a hug would indicate that you agree those desires are valid and worthwhile, and would confirm that you genuinely care about him.

Choice Point 6

You consider responding to Luke in the following ways:

1. Luke makes a good case - time for that hug!
2. Empathically validate Luke's desire for a hug, then share your own perspective about why you will not provide it.
3. Explain why you are unable to hug Luke, but share openly about how important he is to you, and how much you value your relationship.

Discussion

Luke has now explained in some detail why the hug would hold great meaning for him, thus demonstrating a capacity to reflect and not just demand action. Your next step is to empathically validate the sources of his demand ("I can see why a hug would seem to disprove your fears of being rejected") *without* necessarily acting on it. As mentioned earlier, conveying an empathic understanding of patients' emotional predicaments can set the stage for them to reckon more reflectively with the perspective you will now share on the matter. This is important regardless of whether you are unable or unwilling to take the requested action.

Accordingly, the choice to offer validation while also sharing your concerns (Option 2) involves an ideal balance of taking both Luke's perspective and your own perspective seriously. If Luke first feels understood by you, he will be more willing to curiously consider how you reach a different conclusion, while at the same time understanding and validating his emotional needs. Making explicit the departure points between your minds as you reflect together on his wish could help him to re-evaluate his own perspectives on needing concrete proofs of care.

Even after you have achieved some shared understanding about Luke's reasons for wanting a hug, providing it (Option 1) could reinforce his assumption that people only care if they always prove it with action or are willing to cross boundaries. Even just verbally reassuring Luke about his importance to you (Option 3) implies that he requires continued reassurance or an enmeshed relationship to feel okay. In addition to encouraging an unhealthy dependency on your responses to him, these approaches fail to encourage Luke's further reflection about important dynamics unfolding in the therapeutic relationship.

Answers

1. U
2. H
3. U

Principles and Clinical Pearls

1. Once patients are able to elaborate on the emotional meaning of their concrete requests, the therapist should respond by offering genuine empathic validation of patients' perspectives, and then transparently sharing the therapist's own perspective on the situation that is unfolding.

Case Continues...

You say to Luke, "It sounds like this is not just about the hug for you. In our therapy, you've started to desire real closeness with another person. It is really important to you that I acknowledge and value your progress, and a hug from me feels like the only real way for you to trust that I do." Luke responds enthusiastically, "Yes... that's exactly it."

You continue, "I can understand why a hug would have so much meaning for you. But for me it would mean something quite different. For one thing, it would cross a physical boundary that I maintain professionally in all my work. Furthermore, it presumes that physical contact is the only way that you can feel understood or valued by someone. There's something about that that just doesn't sit right with me."

Luke responds introspectively: "Well, when you put it that way, I don't really believe that, either." A deeper discussion ensues about Luke's desire to develop a meaningful romantic connection with another person on multiple levels, not just the physical.

Summary of Clinical Approach

This case highlights multiple forms of nonreflectiveness commonly encountered in work with patients with BPD. Clinicians often feel tempted to employ therapeutic approaches that can inadvertently lead to increased rigidity, disengagement, demandingness, and dependency. Rather, clinicians should aim to stimulate greater reflection and curiosity through a humble and "not-knowing" therapeutic stance, while tailoring their interventions to address the particular forms of nonreflectiveness appearing in the moment. Clinical interventions should be tailored to the distinctive features of particular unreflective states, which can be distinguished as either black-and-white, disconnected, or concrete. For black-and-white thinking, avoid trying to change patients' minds overtly or more discreetly. Instead, empathically validate their perspectives, explore how they arrived at them, and cautiously share your own perspective to stimulate further reflection. For more disconnected experiences, try to "shift the frame" of patients' narratives, either by directing attention to aspects of the here-and-now clinical interaction or through surprising interventions that might abruptly prompt more meaningful reflection. For concrete thinking, avoid the impulse to take concrete action to appease concrete demands. Rather, explore the deeper meaning of patients' demands, empathically validate the underlying emotional experiences, and transparently share your own perspective on the scenario (including any dilemma you feel about "doing" versus "not doing" what is being requested).

Clinician Experience: Surrendering the Expert Role

A common barrier to stimulating meaningful reflection in patients with BPD is our desire to feel like, and present ourselves as, an "expert." In relation to our patients' instability, we may struggle with a range of internal experiences that leave us feeling decidedly "nonexpert." These include insecurities about the quality of our own clinical performance, fear that our patients will never improve, and concerns about how colleagues will evaluate our treatments. We often seek refuge from these experiences by assuming an "expert role" that may entail constantly trying to appear knowledgeable and wise, as though we always have the right answer. Or we may try to *do something* concrete to be helpful, such as teaching cognitive restructuring techniques, coaching behavioral skills, offering advice, or making what we hope will be an insightful interpretation.

These approaches by way of an "expert stance" are often helpful on a variety of levels, but equally often are counterproductive to the goal of stimulating reflection in our patients. They sidestep this goal by relying too heavily upon our own knowledge, competence, and reflection rather than cultivating such processes in the patient.

One safeguard against these errors associated with the "expert stance" is for us to become more attuned to our own impulses to revert to it in particular clinical scenarios. Another is to practice surrendering the expert role altogether when a more "not-knowing" stance would better stimulate patients' reflective capacities. Doing so entails a significant reframing of our role in the therapeutic process. Rather than emphasizing our own knowledge, we focus on the *nature, quality, and outcomes* of our interventions on a moment-to-moment basis, specifically asking to what degree any given intervention increases reflection in our patients.

From this perspective, our sense of competence derives not from how certain we are about what we (or our patients) should do, feel, or think during clinical interactions, but from the extent to which we foster a therapeutic climate in which the patient feels understood well-enough to risk becoming more curious and reflective. Rather than seeing ourselves as authorities holding complete responsibility to create change for patients, we become more like shepherds of a process in which the patient's own mind and reflective capacities are held as the joint focus of therapeutic attention.

To clinicians just beginning to work with BPD, this stance can feel counterintuitive and even negligent, as if we are abandoning our commitment to functional improvement for our patients. However, surrendering the expert stance is not equivalent to indifference about outcomes. On the contrary, one of the major empirically validated treatments for BPD contends that functional improvement is a natural by-product of improving our patients' capacities for inquisitiveness and reflection (see below).

References and Recommendations for Further Reading[1]

1. Bateman A, Fonagy P. Psychotherapy for borderline personality disorder: mentalization-based treatment. Oxford, UK: Oxford University Press; 2004.
2. Bateman A, Fonagy P, editors. Handbook of mentalizing in mental health practice. Washington, D.C.: American Psychiatric Publishing; 2012.
3. Bateman A, Fonagy P. Mentalization-based treatment for personality disorders: a practical guide. Oxford, UK: Oxford University Press; 2016.
4. Choi-Kain LW, Albert EB, Gunderson JG. Evidence-based treatments for borderline personality disorder: implementation, integration, and stepped care. Harv Rev Psychiatry. 2016;24:342–56.
5. Fonagy P, Gergely G, Jurist EL, Target M. Affect regulation, mentalization, and the development of the self. New York: Other Press; 2002.

Robert P. Drozek is an individual and group psychotherapist in the Adult Center for Borderline Personality Disorder at McLean Hospital. He is a teaching associate in the Department of Psychiatry at Harvard Medical School, and a supervisor of Mentalization-Based Treatment through the Anna Freud Centre and McLean's Borderline Personality Disorder Training Institute. He is in private practice in Belmont, Massachusetts.

---

[1] The above ideas are a distillation of the main technical principles of mentalization-based treatment (MBT), one of the major evidence-based treatments for BPD. Mentalization is formally defined as "the mental process by which an individual implicitly and explicitly interprets the actions of herself and others as meaningful on the basis of intentional mental states such as personal desires, needs, feelings, beliefs, and reasons" ([1], p. xxi). More colloquially, mentalizing can be described as "thinking about thinking," "holding mind in mind," and "seeing others from the inside and ourselves from the outside." MBT conceptualizes core BPD-related problems as caused by context-dependent impairments in mentalizing, such that, when patients are under increased interpersonal stress, they are more at risk for all of the nonreflective processes considered in this chapter. The treatment model provides accessible strategies to stimulate patients' mentalizing processes in the clinical moment. This work over time helps to strengthen patients' reflection on their thoughts and emotions in the context of their relationships, resulting in improvements in BPD's characteristic instabilities in emotions, self-esteem, relationships, and behavior. For further information about MBT, see the publications listed below, and especially the comprehensive treatment manual [3].

Approach to Suicidal Behaviors

Igor Weinberg

Choice Point Index
1. Responding to "provocative" suicidal statements
2. Addressing rapid resolution of suicidal urges
3. Suicidal urges used to elicit greater support
4. Suicide in the setting of hopelessness in an ongoing treatment
5. Consideration of clinician experience in the discussion of suicide

Introduction

A lifetime history of suicide attempts is reported by 46–70% (median = 65%; Zanarini et al.), and completed suicide becomes the tragic end for 3–10% (median = 5%; [12, 18]) of BPD patients. Typically, these patients have a history of multiple attempts [18]. Not surprisingly, such suicidal behaviors in BPD patients are a common reason that clinicians experience trepidation, reluctance, and antagonism when they consider taking these patients into their clinical practices [2]. But avoiding psychiatric patients that might kill themselves is similar to refusing care to cancer patient because of their high mortality rate. A more effective way of dealing with this – quite realistic – anxiety is to receive training in treatment of these patients. Clinicians who receive psycho-education on BPD or training in its treatment report improved attitude and empathy to these patients [6, 7, 15, 16].

In the last two decades, a number of treatments demonstrated effectiveness in reducing suicide risk in BPD patients. The research shows that BPD can be effectively treated [14], and suicidality in BPD generally improves over the course of treatment [19]. Typically, suicide risk significantly decreases in the first 6 months of

I. Weinberg, Ph.D.
McLean Hospital/Harvard Medical School, Belmont, MA, USA
e-mail: iweinberg@mclean.harvard.edu

© Springer International Publishing AG, part of Springer Nature 2018
B. Palmer, B. Unruh (eds.), *Borderline Personality Disorder*,
https://doi.org/10.1007/978-3-319-90743-7_3

intervention and continues to further diminish as the treatment progresses. Most treatments demonstrate similar degrees of effectiveness, though Mentalization-Based Treatment (MBT) seems to be slightly more effective than Dialectical Behavior Therapy (DBT), Cognitive Behavior Therapy (CBT), or psychodynamic therapies [19]. This is consistent with the findings that most effective treatments for suicidality in BPD share a number of commonalities, including treatment frame, suicidality management strategies, attention to affect, proactive therapists, and exploratory/change-oriented interventions [20, 21].

Case 1

Annabel is a 30-year-old single woman who started treatment in a partial hospital program. She came 45 min late to the admission interview for the program, excusing her tardiness by blaming an "impossible mother" she "had to talk to." Her loud voice, abundance of makeup, and profuse gesticulation complemented her use of dramatic language, such as: "always," "never," "the best," and "the worst." Once the admission interview has gotten off the ground, she proceeded to ask the admitting psychiatrist – a resident in psychiatric training – if she can be given some evidence or proof that the program is indeed helpful. She indicated that if not, she might as well kill herself.

Choice Point

For each intervention, choose H: "helpful," U: "unhelpful or harmful," or P: "perhaps helpful, with reservations."
    How would the psychiatrist best respond to that comment?

1. Hospitalize the patient to contain suicide risk and evaluate her further, given her apparent functional difficulties (lateness) and suicidal plan (to kill herself if the program does not help).
2. Conduct a detailed chain analysis identifying reasons that led her to think about suicide.
3. Interpret that her suicide is misdirected aggression against her mother (murder in 180 degrees), following their difficult interaction that morning.
4. Offer an "irreverent comment" that suicide is a choice and that there is absolutely no evidence that this program helps dead people

Discussion

This is an example of one particular type of suicidal behaviors – suicide threats. It is common in patients with comorbid histrionic or narcissistic features and has been found to be related to interpersonal needs, rather than communication of the suicidal intent *per se* [3]. Most commonly the patient is testing the clinician ("Does he or she care?"), seeking attention or care — especially if they are uncertain whether the clinician cares — or expressing anger if the patient believes the clinician does not care. Effective responding to such communications will engage Annabel, while ineffective communication is likely to alienate her or iatrogenically reinforce suicidality and nonproductive engagement. For example, response 1 is a likely response to a patient who is communicating *a bona fide* imminent suicide plan. However, Annabel is not communicating a plan, nor she is indicating an imminent risk. This type of response will not allow engagement to occur – it is likely to only decrease the clinician's anxiety with a risk of communicating rejection to the patient. Response 2 is a conservative option, though in this context, it takes the mention of suicide as if the patient intends it as a communication, not a strategic maneuver in the dialogue with the clinician. It risks iatrogenically reinforcing the "suicide talk" by teaching that suicidal comments elicit greater caring and concern than direct emotional expression (such as describing her fear about starting a new program). Some patients might see that response as an indication that the therapist cares, especially if they feel as if the more the therapist does, the more he or she cares. Response 3 is least likely to be helpful and most likely to make the patient feel misunderstood. While such interpretations may be accurate, they confuse and anger patients who might not have the capacity to immediately see the relevance of such dynamics to their behavior. Response 4 is likely to match Annabel's otherwise dramatic style. It is likely to avoid the risk of reinforcing "suicide talk" by not colluding with the intention to elicit caring responses upon which patients may come to depend. Following irreverent responses with curiosity about what elicited the suicide comments, with an eye toward naming her fear that she will not feel helpfully supported, would make a very effective intervention.

Answers

1. U
2. P
3. U
4. H

Case 2

Melody is a 24-year-old woman who was rushed into emergency room following a distressed call to 911 by her family. Melody took "all the pills" in the medicine cabinet after Brian – the love of her life – announced a much-feared breakup earlier that day. They have been seeing each other on and off for a couple of years. Melody was hoping to marry Brian, though Brian was reluctant to propose given her spotty employment history and bad temper. Melody described a tendency to drink alcohol or order large amounts of takeout food to soothe her anxiety about their relationship. Two days after the admission, Brian visited her on the unit and the couple decided to "try again." Delighted, Melody asked to see the unit's psychiatrist, requesting early discharge because her "crisis and suicidality have successfully resolved."

Choice Points

How should the inpatient psychiatrist respond to Melody's request for immediate discharge?

1. Melody can be discharged because she is no longer suicidal and happily reunited with Brian.
2. Melody can be discharged and referred to couple's counseling because her suicidality is a by-product of this couple's dynamics.
3. The psychiatrist can validate the relief that Melody feels, then engage her in a discussion regarding the function of her suicide attempt and whether she would like to address her tendency to use suicide as a solution for relational issues.
4. The psychiatrist should refuse to discharge the patient because he or she "needs to get more information to evaluate that decision."

Suicide attempts in the context of interpersonal drama are common in BPD patients. This is the most typical scenario encountered by clinicians in these patients. The couple's reunion, while surprising and dramatic, is not uncommon either. Research shows that suicide attempts in fact lead to increased social support [23], though this is not an effective long-term solution. One problem is that significant others may feel coerced or manipulated into providing support, as Brian may feel around the reunion here. This creates an unsustainable relational dynamic. Response #1 is the one that Melody suggests herself. It minimizes suicide as a problem and misattributes the problem to the breakup, as opposed to Melody's use of suicide as a solution. The issue is to help Melody shift toward learning about her suicidal process and ways to intervene more effectively when the situation repeats. Suggesting couples counseling (response #2) does not solve the problem of using suicide as a solution (it frames couples issues as the problem instead), and it does not enlist the patient in taking ownership over her problems and her treatment. Response #3 offers the most effective way to engage Melody in treatment. Validation offers a very powerful starting point in helping Melody recognize that her current experience of relief occurs within the context of a powerful interpersonal pattern in which her suicidal statements may be pulling Brian back in, but ultimately destabilize their relationship. Response #4 is "technically" right – it gives a good reason as to why discharge is premature. However, when presented that way it misses the opportunity to assist the patient in contextualizing her current emotional reality.

Answers

1. U
2. P
3. H
4. U

Case 3

Delilah is a 28-year-old woman who was attending an intensive outpatient DBT program. In her treatment, she was addressing nonsuicidal cutting and developed a pattern of calling her therapist for coaching, lying about her level of distress in order to prolong the phone contact, and thereby eliciting desired validation and interpersonal contact. She described her therapist as "the perfect replacement" for her mother and was hoping that by increased contact with her she could "make up" for repeated failings of her mother during childhood. The same evening that Delilah's therapist left for a brief vacation, Delilah proceeded to the local emergency room, indicating that she feels "unsafe" and that she might do "something irreversible." Delilah mentioned that her therapist will be "mad" to find out that she went to emergency room and did not use skills or call the covering therapist instead.

Choice Points

How should the ER clinician manage Delilah's presentation?

1. Delilah should be hospitalized to further assess risk and to be "on the safe side."
2. Delilah should be hospitalized on the unit that she dislikes and given only minimal privileges to make the inpatient experience more aversive.
3. The ER clinician should communicate the situation to the covering clinician, encourage Delilah to get in touch with him or her, and not admit Delilah to the inpatient unit.
4. The ER clinician can describe the dilemma: "Of course I can hospitalize you, but would that really help you or actually harm you by reinforcing use of suicide to get your interpersonal needs met?" Discussion of the dilemma can then lead to hospitalization or discharge from the ER.
5. The ER clinician should ask Delilah to use behavioral skills to self-regulate while she is in ER and postpone any admission decision until the skills work or do not.
6. The ER clinician can offer an interpretation that Delilah is angry at her therapist who made her feel abandoned and therefore now has the urge to harm the treatment.

This is a common dilemma with suicidal BPD patients. This case demonstrates one of the scenarios that may make clinicians reluctant to take such patients into their practices – reporting suicidality in the context of a therapist's imperfect availability. This case also demonstrates a number of responses that can be helpful in using the suicide crisis productively. Understanding Delilah's behavior in the context of frantic efforts to elicit care from her environment through escalation of distress-associated behaviors should guide the management of the current ER visit. The goal is to recognize this dynamic, name it, and make the response to it nonreinforcing. Response #1 is conservative and in the service of the clinician's anxiety. This response is likely what Delilah is aiming for with her tentative presentation of her suicidal threat ("might do something unsafe"). It is likely to reinforce the pattern of the behavior, though it is frequently used in clinical practice out of undue and unhelpful caution. In this case, documentation of pros vs. cons of the assessment and level of care determination, consultation with a colleague, and discussion of the situation with the outpatient clinician can protect from medico-legal risks and from the risk of iatrogenesis. Response #2 is mixed in value – it gives with one hand (offers the desired hospitalization) and takes away with the other (makes it not rewarding) but may be perceived as passive–aggressive and minimizes the patient's capacity to meaningfully participate in the decision. The reality of implementing such decision requires an outpatient team prepared to refer the patient to a particular unit, and an inpatient team willing to accept a difficult patient and "hold the line" regarding the conditions of the admission. Response #3 helpfully redirects Delilah to her outpatient therapy and enlists her in a proactive role. Response #4 – also known as "Principle of False Submission" [4] helps shift the discussion to the functions of suicidality away from the binary negotiation of getting hospitalized or not. Response #5 is a possibility, though is likely to backfire if Delilah decides to make the case that "skills do not work" and reports lack of improvement in the service of getting hospitalized. Response #6 is an interpretation and is likely to anger Delilah who might not have the capacity to make use of such an abstract intervention.

Answers

1. U
2. U
3. P
4. H
5. P
6. P

Case 4

Geoff is a 40-year-old single man who was seeing his therapist for over 5 years. In course of his treatment, he made some noticeable progress. Initially, he was unsure whether or not he wanted to stay alive, he was employed outside area of his area of training, and he was completely isolated. In course of treatment, he made a commitment to staying alive, worked on life-related goals ("build a life worth living"), found a job related to his training as yoga instructor, and consequently doubled his salary as well as started making time to spend with friends. For a while, things were "looking up," and Geoff was reporting satisfaction in moving toward these goals. On occasion, Geoff would report intense feelings of jealousy and sadness realizing that all his friends have been "coupled up" and he was "lonely and perpetually single." He reported that his last romantic relationship ended a decade ago, right before he developed a suicidal depression, lost his yoga studio, and went on to receive multiple courses of ECT before he got better. He remained single ever since, feeling embarrassed over his lost career. Invariable these acute crises would "resolve" and Geoff would de-prioritize romantic life over his work. One day, he reported a plan to go away for a vacation to the family house. He reported that he was really looking forward to it because "all I am doing is working." As the discussion of the vacation plan progressed, the therapist discovered that Geoff in fact planned to isolate himself during the vacation and kill himself by taking the pills that he had accumulated in the preceding months. The therapist was shocked by this unexpected revelation of suicidality, because otherwise Geoff had seemed to be engaged in treatment, attached to the therapist, and making progress.

Choice Points

How should the therapist respond to Geoff's sudden disclosure of a suicide plan?

1. As the patient seems engaged in therapy and attached to the therapist, the therapist can manage the crisis on an outpatient basis and hope that the therapeutic attachment will protect the patient from suicide.
2. As the patient failed to disclose the plan on his own and in advance, this constitutes violation of the prior commitment to therapy, thus the therapy should be terminated and Geoff needs to be hospitalized.
3. The therapist should first help Geoff in getting hospitalized, then facilitate a discussion while Geoff is in a more contained setting of what led to the suicidal thinking and nondisclosure of it in treatment.
4. The therapist needs to ask Geoff to sign a suicide contract and develop a safety plan, then let Geoff go to the much desired vacation but conduct daily check-ins on the telephone to ensure his safety.
5. The therapist should request a consultation from a colleague to assess Geoff, the treatment, and the need for further intervention/hospitalization.

This case describes a recurrence of *a bona fide* suicidality in otherwise improving patient. Studies report that midlife crises are especially difficult for BPD patients who start coming to terms with missed opportunities or experience significant losses [9]. This is one of the reasons that the risk of serious planned suicidality increases with age [24], even though the risk of impulsive suicidality diminishes with age [25]. This case also exemplifies a number of important aspects of suicidality in BPD patients: (1) Suicidality in these patients sometimes develops independently of major depressive disorder [24]. Depression is not a precondition for such suicidality, even though the patient can be as serious about planning, intending, and executing the suicide as the most lethal depressed patients. (2) Patients are likely to have deficits in disclosure of suicidality [1]. Sometimes the deficits are related to difficulty reporting it to clinician (due to shame or not wanting the clinician to interfere with execution of suicide) and sometimes they are due to limitations in self-awareness (due to dissociation/splitting or alexithymia). (3) Lack of attention to patient's sexual and romantic life are commonly found in histories of patients that killed themselves during treatment [5]. This indicates that recurrent feelings of distress that Geoff experienced around singleness required more significant attention, despite his tendency to minimize that subject.

Response #1 counts on the assumption that therapeutic relationship can sustain patients through difficult times, including suicidal crises. Though true in some cases, therapeutic relationship cannot sustain every patient and not in every suicidal crisis [22]. With Geoff, it did not protect him from planning the suicide – an ominous sign that the relationship with the therapist is not sufficient. Response #2 is an example of punitive countertransference mistake. Violation of rules is a clinical reality that can be learned from, not reasons for terminating treatment that became more demanding. Response #3 is likely to contain the risk of acting on a suicidal plan and invites the patient to examine reasons for his suicidal plan along with reasons for not sharing suicidality in treatment. It takes some persistence and art to convince the patient to agree to a voluntary admission. Response #4 relies too much on self-report of the patient, as opposed to understanding of the suicidal dynamics, and overestimates the power of safety contracts and daily check-ins. Safety contracts have no empirical support of effectively increasing collaboration with the clinician and thus reducing risk of suicide [13]. When patients decide to die, they are not likely to care about such contract. Response #5, if available and practical, may be appropriate. A colleague would likely be able to further assess Geoff's commitment to suicide and the gaps that his treatment has failed to meaningfully address but may be fueling his suicidal thinking. It serves a similar function to Response #3 (additional eyes, taking the patient's concern seriously) without the safety that is inherent in immediate hospitalization (but would not preclude hospitalization if the colleague agreed).

Answers

1. U
2. U
3. H
4. U
5. H

Case 5

Fernando is a 35-year-old divorced man who came to his regular outpatient therapy appointment. His therapy was helping him with his bad temper, angry outbursts that result in broken doors and cell phones as well as bouts of heavy drinking. His ex-wife – Christina – filed for divorce when he lost his fifth job in a row due to his emotional volatility that intimidated his customers. Since then, he has been working odd jobs and contemplated numerous plans for how to get Christina back. During the appointment, Fernando appeared despondent, slowed down, and reluctantly reported that he was considering killing himself since he woke up in the morning.

Choice Points

How should the clinician respond to Fernando's suicidal statements and affective presentation?

1. Clinician should say: "I would not worry about these feelings – they will pass soon. How is your new job going?"
2. Clinician should say: "Thank you for letting me know – let me call your psychopharmacologist so we can decide what to do."
3. Clinician should say: "You must be thinking of killing yourself because you cannot get Christina back."
4. Clinician should file for involuntary commitment to inpatient unit.
5. Clinician should say: "Can you tell me what was on your mind when you started thinking about killing yourself?"

Suicidality provokes strong feelings in clinicians [8, 11]. These feelings are not easy to bear. Consequently, many clinicians react to suicidal crisis using whatever coping strategy they adapt in their personal life to cope with intense feelings, such as fears of loss, despair, anger, loss of control – to name just a few. These result in different types of misguided interventions (see Sidebar). The art of suicide intervention with Fernando is meeting him where he is at and helping him articulate, share, and ultimately bear feelings of despair, loss, and shame. This is an arduous task for a therapist, and different responses exemplify various defensive postures against emotional engagement with Fernando (responses #1–4), whereas response #5 invites Fernando to elaborate on his internal experience – a response that is more in line with the life-saving emotional engagement, attachment, and reflectiveness.

Answers

1. U
2. U
3. U

4. U
5. H

Summary of Clinical Approach

Suicide, suicide attempts, suicidal thoughts and plans, and suicidal communications are common in BPD. The overarching treatment goal is to help the patient shift from repeating suicidal processes to trying to understand and change them – making painful thoughts, feelings, and urges both more evident and more manageable. This process is complicated by clinician reactions and the many possible uses of suicidal communications. The process of recognizing and accurately assessing risk, while maintaining attention to interpersonal dynamics and the patient's subjective experience [17], can help ground clinicians and contribute to effective care.

Clinical Errors in Responding to Suicidal Patients [10]

Superficial reassurance
Avoidance of strong feelings
Hiding behind professionalism
Inadequate suicide assessment
Failure to identify suicide precipitating event
Passivity
Insufficient directiveness
Advice giving
Defensiveness
Stereotypical responses

References

1. Apter A, Horesh N, Gothelf D, Graffi H, Lepkifker E. Relationship between self-disclosure and serious suicidal behavior. Compr Psychiatry. 2001;42(1):70–5.
2. Bodner E, Cohen-Fridel S, Iancu I. Staff attitudes towards patients with borderline personality disorder. Compr Psychiatry. 2011;52(5):548–55.
3. García-Nieto R, Blasco-Fontecilla H, de León-Martinez V, Baca-García E. Clinical features associated with suicide attempts versus suicide gestures in an inpatient sample. Arch Suicide Res. 2014;18(4):419–31.
4. Gunderson JG. Good psychiatric management of borderline personality disorder. Washington, DC: American Psychiatric Publishing; 2008.
5. Hendin H, Haas AP, Maltsberger JT, Koestner B, Szanto K. Problems in psychotherapy with suicidal patients. Am J Psychiatry. 2006;163(1):67–72.
6. Keuroghlian AS, Palmer BA, Choi-Kain LW, Borba CP, Links PS, Gunderson JG. The effect of attending good psychiatric management (GPM) workshops on attitudes toward patients with borderline personality disorder. J Personal Disord. 2016;30(4):567–76.

7. Knaak S, Szeto AC, Fitch K, Modgill G, Patten S. Stigma towards borderline personality disorder: effectiveness and generalizability of an anti-stigma program for healthcare providers using a pre-post randomized design. Borderline Personal Disord Emot Dysregul. 2015;2:9.
8. Maltsberger JT, Buie DH. (1974). Countertransference hate in the treatment of suicidal patients. Arch Gen Psychiatry. 1974 May;30(5):625–33.
9. McGlashan T. The chestnut lodge follow-up study. III Long-term outcome of borderline personalities. Arch Gen Psychiatry. 1986;43(1):20–30.
10. Neimeyer RA, Pfeffer AM. The ten most common errors of suicide prevention. In: Leenaars AA, Maltesberg JT, Neimeyer RA, editors. Washington, DC: Taylor & Francis. Treatment of suicidal people; 1994. p. 207–24.
11. Orbach I. Therapeutic empathy with the suicidal wish: principles of therapy with suicidal individuals. Am J Psychother. 2001;55(2):166–84.
12. Pompili M, Girardi P, Ruberto A, Tatarelli R. Suicide in borderline personality disorder: a meta-analysis. Nord J Psychiatry. 2005;59(5):319–24.
13. Rudd MD, Mandrusiak M, Joiner TE Jr. The case against no-suicide contracts: the commitment to treatment statement as a practice alternative. J Clin Psychol. 2006;62(2):243–51.
14. Stoffers JM, Völlm BA, Rücker G, Timmer A, Huband N, Lieb K. Psychological therapies for people with borderline personality disorder. Cochrane Database Syst Rev. 2012;(8):CD005652.
15. Shanks C, Pfohl B, Blum N, Black DW. Can attitudes towards patients with borderline personality disorder be changed? The effects of attending a STEPPS workshop. J Personal Disord. 2011;25(6):806–12.
16. Warrender D. Staff nurse perceptions of the impact of mentalization-based therapy skills training when working with borderline personality disorder in acute mental health: a qualitative study. J Psychiatr Ment Health Nurs. 2015;22:623–33.
17. Weinberg, I. Taxonomy of suicidal behaviors in borderline personality disorder. 2nd international congress on borderline personality disorder; Amsterdam; 2012.
18. Weinberg I, Maltsberger JT. Suicidal behaviors in borderline personality disorder. In: Suicide in psychiatric disorders. New York: Nova Editorial Inc.; 2007. p. 333–70.
19. Weinberg I, Richman M. Meta-analysis of treatment outcome studies for suicide attempts in BPD. In: 3d congress of the north American Society for Study of personality disorders. Boston: MA; 2015.
20. Weinberg I, Ronningstam E, Goldblatt MJ Schechter M, Wheelis J, Maltsberger JT. Strategies in treatment of suicidality: identification of common and treatment-specific interventions in empirically supported treatment manuals. J Clin Psychiatry. 2010;71(6):699–706.
21. Weinberg I, Ronningstam E, Goldblatt MJ Schechter M, Maltsberger JT. Common factors in empirically supported treatments of borderline personality disorder. CurrPsychiatry Rep. 2011;13(1):60–8.
22. Weinberg I, Ronningstam E, Goldblatt MJ, Maltsberger JT. Vicissitudes of the therapeutic alliance with suicidal patients: a psychoanalytic perspective. In: Michel K, Jobes D, editors. Building a therapeutic alliance with the suicidal patient. Washington DC: APA; 2010. p. 293–316.
23. Walker RL, Joiner TE Jr, Rudd MD. The course of post-crisis suicidal symptoms: how and for whom is suicide "cathartic"? Suicide Life Threat Behav. 2001;31(2):144–52.
24. Soloff PH, Fabio A, Kelly TM, Malone KM, Mann JJ. High-lethality status in patients with borderline personality disorder. J Personal Disord. 2005;19(4):386–99.
25. Zanarini MC, Frankenburg FR, Reich DB, Fitzmaurice G, Weinberg I, Gunderson JG. The 10-year course of physically self-destructive acts reported by borderline patients and axis II comparison subjects. Acta Psychiatr Scand. 2008;117(3):177–84.

Dr. Weinberg was born in Moscow, former USSR, and immigrated to Israel in his teens. He completed Ph.D. in clinical psychology, studying suicide and came to McLean Hospital where he continued to specialize in using evidence-based treatments for suicidal patients with personality disorders. He published empirical, review, and clinical papers in peer-review journals and delivered conference presentations and workshops on treatment of suicidal patients with personality disorders.

Navigating Intersession Contact

4

Karen Jacob

Case Introduction

Jane is a 28-year-old single Caucasian woman who sought treatment with you several weeks ago due to ongoing difficulties in intimate relationships causing her to feel more alone, desperate, and sad. In response to her feelings of despair, she reported a history of cutting, overdosing, abusing substances, and an interpersonal pattern of "lashing out" with threats when hurt or upset in a relationship. Just prior to beginning treatment with you, she found herself managing a complicated legal situation prompted by sending a threatening text to her partner following an argument. This was the latest of many relationships destroyed by her volatility, and she finally felt worn down by her own impulsivity as she yearned for a partner and a family of her own. She wanted to use treatment to better understand her own vulnerabilities and more effectively regulate and express her emotions without destroying relationships.

K. Jacob, Ph.D.
Gunderson Residence, McLean Hospital, Belmont, MA, USA

Department of Psychiatry, Harvard Medical School, Cambridge, MA, USA
e-mail: Kjacob@mclean.harvard.edu

© Springer International Publishing AG, part of Springer Nature 2018
B. Palmer, B. Unruh (eds.), *Borderline Personality Disorder*,
https://doi.org/10.1007/978-3-319-90743-7_4

Your initial assessment revealed a long history of feeling overlooked and dismissed by her parents. They felt overwhelmed by professional obligations before she was born, and her arrival increased their marital distress. They coped by immersing themselves in their jobs until the marriage ended in divorce just as Jane was entering elementary school. She struggled due to having minimal support from either parent and felt very isolated, taking solace in playing alone with her toys and busying herself with activities. As she entered adolescence, she found herself increasingly enraged at her parents and turned to substances to quell her anger. She blamed her academic and social disappointments on her parents and would explode at them in fits of rage until they could no longer abide these outbursts and sent her to boarding school.

Jane navigated the remainder of her early life relatively successfully and without incident, but her anger toward her parents persisted and she avoided returning home to see them. When she sought treatment with you, she claimed that she had learned to accept her parents as flawed and likely unchangeable, and though she continued to harbor resentment toward them, she did not want to engage in family therapy as she was relatively self-sufficient with only minimal contact with them. You suggested that her parents seek psycho-education about BPD through family connections. Jane reluctantly allowed you to make this recommendation and was surprised, though uncomfortable, to hear they seemed eager to learn about BPD and ways they could be more supportive of her.

At the outset of your work with Jane, you discuss the proposed treatment frame and its expectations of her. She had previously been treated by a dialectical behavior therapy (DBT) therapist who made herself available for frequent intersession contact. Jane assumed that your availability would be similar and demanded that you be responsive if needed during this critical time when she would be acclimating to a new therapist and had agreed to allow her parents an unprecedented level of involvement in her treatment.

Choice Point 1

For each intervention, choose H: "helpful," U: "unhelpful or harmful," or P: "perhaps helpful, with reservations."

Regarding Jane's demands, would you:

1. Inquire about the reasons for her demands, to elicit further clarification.
2. Regardless of the reasons for her requests, set firm limits prohibiting any intersession contact.
3. Validate her wish for you to be more available and negotiate terms of intersession contact.
4. Refer her back to a DBT therapist given her need for coaching and tell her to return to you once she feels ready to suspend intersession contact.
5. Validate her reasons for requesting increased availability and explain that you will not prohibit intersession contact, but your availability is inherently limited and her reasons for contacting you between sessions should be explored in the treatment.

Discussion

Treatment is off to a good start, and Jane expressed feeling understood by you but is fearful that she will need more support than you have alluded to providing during the initial phase of the treatment. You recognize that she is feeling very alone in the world and perhaps threatened by having her parents get involved in family connections as their change may leave her feeling more exposed and vulnerable. You want to support her for expressing her concerns about this directly and in words (not actions), in an effort to preempt her typical explosions. If you ignore her requests, you may be inadvertently reinforcing her perceived need to "show you" in actions (not words this time) that she cannot manage herself more independently. Thus, this frame-setting conversation presents a typical early opportunity to shape future behavior by appreciating her attempts to communicate her wishes verbally. However, offering availability that goes beyond your typical treatment frame could inadvertently reinforce her anxiety about her capacities by communicating, either implicitly or explicitly, that you agree she cannot manage in between sessions.

You choose to praise her direct request for help while gently reminding her that treatment is geared toward promoting her independence. You share your faith in her that, despite her fears, she can manage on her own in most circumstances, and you promise to do your best to be available to help if true emergencies arise.

Answers

1. H
2. U
3. P
4. P
5. H

Principles and Clinical Pearls

1. Setting expectations and parameters around intersession contact early on creates a valuable platform for framing the larger focus and goals of treatment around enhancing patients' independence over time.
2. Patients generally feel contained not only by hearing they may try to reach you in emergencies but also by hearing there are some predictable ways in which you will not be available due to inherent limitations on your own time and capacity to be helpful to them.
3. Taking the time to listen to patients' concerns about needing more support and explain your rationale for limiting intersession availability allows for important early alliance building through validation of patients' previous experiences and expressing your belief in their capacities to grow and change over the course of treatment.

4. Many BPD patients initially report great difficulty managing themselves independently between sessions, or would prefer to have a more dependent therapeutic relationship. This is not sufficient reason to offer more involved intersession contact or to refer them elsewhere. Only if you assess that your patient truly cannot manage a basic level of safety during an initial phase of treatment should you consider offering the more intensive alternative of DBT, which formally includes intersession coaching as a core treatment element.

Case Continues...

You begin working with Jane, and she agrees to family involvement via psychoeducation. As part of your treatment plan, you also share your expectation that she continues to work at a job. You stress the importance of creating a predictable, structured daily life routine as a more stable functional platform from which she can better address her longstanding relationship issues. You also recommend that she suspend dating for the first few months to cultivate more independence and focus on stabilizing her relationship with her parents. You predict that her family's increased involvement will re-expose her to challenging interpersonal dynamics she has long avoided, and that these relationships warrant initial focus given her continued emotional and financial dependency on her parents.

Jane is eager to continue her current part-time job at a department store. Although she finds interpersonal tensions with colleagues challenging, she feels valued by the company for her persuasive powers and top sales performance and recognizes that this is an important source of mastery and competence. However, she protests your recommendation that she suspend dating and tells you that she will agree to this for a short time because she wants to work with you but adds that she will not adhere to this recommendation long-term due to her interest in finding a partner and starting a family. During your session on a Thursday afternoon, she reminds you that her biological clock is ticking as she nears age 30, and worries that she will never move forward toward building her own family.

Two days later on Saturday night, you receive an urgent call from Jane at 11:30 PM. Given that she has thus far followed your agreement to have no intersession contact, you imagine she may be experiencing an unusual amount of distress and decide to answer. She blurts out that she is feeling suicidal and unsure of how to keep herself safe. You inquire about what prompted this situation and learn that she has been dating a man she met 3 weeks prior who broke up with her over dinner this very evening.

Choice Point 2

With regard to Jane's crisis call, how do you respond?

1. Share your disappointment that she diverted from your agreement to suspend dating and say that you will speak to her during your next session about the problems in the therapy.

2. Direct her to an emergency room for safety evaluation and get off of the phone as quickly as possible, given that this situation has arisen due to her breaching a treatment agreement.
3. Validate that she is understandably upset about the loss of this relationship given her interests in finding a partner, and then redirect her to an emergency room.
4. Validate her feelings of rejection and ask her to make a plan for herself to manage her behavioral responses to an understandably difficult situation. You also share your concerns about her electing to date without telling you, given your explicit agreement to defer romantic relationships during your early work together.
5. You validate her feelings and remind her that she has proven herself capable of managing several breakups in the past. You remind her that she can always visit the emergency room if she continues to struggle, but express your hope that she will manage to keep herself safe as you are hoping to see her for her next scheduled appointment in a few days. You do not raise the issue of her breaching treatment expectations over the phone, but intend to do so in person at her next session.

Discussion

BPD treatments cannot work without honesty and transparency. Yet patients often depart from treatment recommendations even after expressing agreement with the plan and rationale you initially outlined, then once the departure comes to light may defensively justify their wish to follow their own plan. Patients' reasons for deviating from explicitly agreed upon recommendations are important to explore, but you should do so during scheduled sessions even if you learn the deviation during an intersession crisis. If your patient is contacting you in a crisis stemming from a hidden deviation from treatment agreements, the top priority is to appreciate and reinforce her honesty and then help manage her current difficulties, including making a plan for safety that emphasizes not only available emergency resources but also your hope that she will manage herself safely so you can see her as soon as possible at the next scheduled session. Maintaining a supportive, problem-solving stance during the crisis call while appreciating any steps taken toward greater transparency in that moment can foster an environment in which treatment deviations can be more openly discussed at the next session. At the next session, it helps empathize with patients' difficulty adhering to recommendations while restating their relevance to her own long-term treatment goals.

Answers

1. U
2. U
3. U
4. P
5. H

Principles and Clinical Pearls

1. BPD patients often enter treatment with the explicit goal of wanting a romantic relationship. But given their profound interpersonal vulnerabilities, most treatment approaches discourage patients from entering into intimate relationships during the early stages of treatment to stabilize in other, less activating areas of life. Therapists can help patients to better manage the inevitable vicissitudes of romantic partnerships by emphasizing the need to first build a more stable functional baseline. Good psychiatric management for BPD, a basic treatment approach that is easily employed by clinicians without special expertise in BPD, strongly recommends that patients establish stable work prior to seeking out love relationships [1]. The latter are more triggering of abandonment fears and experiences of real or perceived rejection which easily send patients reeling into states of distress accompanied by significant behavioral reactivity [2].

2. Rapid and rigid perceptions of abandonment and rejection are more common early in treatment when BPD patients lack the self-awareness, skill, or experience needed to process nuances in close relationships without making assumptions incompatible with their partners' actual intentions [3]. Given longstanding expectations and fears that people will leave them, patients are primed to react to even minor indications of disinterest, and by assuming, rejection is inevitable and imminent, contributing to the early demise of relationships.

Case Continues...

You see Jane the following week and she has reconstituted since her crisis call. She expresses shame for having hidden this relationship from you and for not being more capable of entering into an intimate relationship at this time in her life. She explains that she understood the reasons for your recommendation but felt acutely desperate to find a partner and fearful that her time is running out. She reminds you that all she wants in this life is to find love, so putting relationships on the backburner feels unbearable to her. You express your understanding of her immense anxiety arising from your recommendation as well as her own long history of romantic difficulties prior to ever seeing you. You then remind her that her past relationships have failed partly due to her longstanding interpersonal vulnerabilities, emotional sensitivity, behavioral reactivity, and fragile sense of self. You share your concern that close relationships are likely to remain challenging for her until these vulnerabilities are stabilized through achieving greater independence and learning to more effectively manage relationships with less at stake, such as with coworkers and friends. With all this in mind, she recommits to deferring dating for the first 3 months of your work together.

Treatment progresses and your conversation about transparency proves useful, as Jane becomes more forthcoming about her desires to date while remaining committed to first working on herself and on relationships with colleagues, friends, and family. However, she often finds herself feeling very alone, even when she is at a family gathering or with a larger crowd of colleagues or friends. She is very anxious and highly self-critical of her interactions in these social situations. She increasingly limits her contact with others and races home from work to spend most evenings and weekends by herself. She reports growing anxiety and depression and less interest in pursuing activities outside of work. You share with her your observations and concern that minimizing social exposure is only causing her to feel worse. You suggest that she works against her fear to increase her activities outside of treatment and work. She identifies several activities that she is willing to pursue during the next week including yoga class, dinner with colleagues during the week, and movie night with childhood friends over the upcoming weekend. You express enthusiasm for these plans while and help her elaborate challenges she may experience. She expresses her desire to follow through with her plan.

The weekend arrives, and Jane contacts you multiple times on Friday, then again on Saturday. You are responsive to her calls and texts given your awareness of her anxieties related to increase her social activities. However, you observe that the frequency of her contact is increasing, and you begin to fear that she is becoming overly dependent on you to help her manage her anxiety. You worry that you may be inadvertently reinforcing a dependency she previously had displayed with romantic partners. You have this in mind when she contacts you again on Sunday as she is driving to her yoga class.

Choice Point 3

How would you respond to Jane's call on Sunday?

1. You answer the phone and you tell her that she is doing a wonderful job. You commend her for following through with all of her weekend plans thus far and cheerlead her toward carrying out her Sunday plans.
2. You reluctantly answer the phone and inquire about the reasons for her call. She predictably shares that she is once again anxious, and you tell her you are concerned that she is reaching out to you again because you had already reviewed a plan with her during your last in-person session. You refer her back to your outlined plan and tell her that you will see her at her next session.
3. You decide to not answer the phone as you realize that your prior phone conversations with her on Friday and Saturday were not crisis driven and plan to take this up with her when you see her during your next session.
4. You answer the phone, and she reports paralyzing anxiety that she will not be able to follow through with her yoga class. You validate her concerns and remind her of past successes, as recently as yesterday. You sense her desire to keep you on the phone but end the call by reminding her of her capacities to self-regulate and your wish to see her soon to further explore her current difficulties. You make a note to yourself to discuss the function of her intersession contact further during your next session.

Discussion

BPD patients exhibit a propensity toward becoming overly dependent on therapists to help them manage issues they need to learn to manage on their own. Increasing dependency within a treatment often appears in the form of escalating intersession contact. Among several empirically validated treatments for BPD, only some specifically encourage intersession contact with patients. Dialectical behavioral therapy (DBT) posits that many patients require "skills coaching" by phone or text in between sessions to learn and implement more effective strategies to manage their lives and curb self-destructive tendencies [4, 5].

Although DBT is demonstrably an effective treatment for helping patients to increase self-awareness, emotion regulation, and behavioral control, treatments that encourage intersession contact for patients present unique clinical challenges [6]. Given that BPD patients have specific difficulties tolerating and managing dependency within close relationships, intersession contact may facilitate overreliance on the therapist and a range of difficult feelings in response to feeling overly dependent [2]. When parameters around intersession contact are not clearly established and consistently followed, therapists run the risk of inadvertently reinforcing dependency that runs counter to treatment goals (choice 4). Consistency with the "rules" of intersession contact can help both the patient and the therapist understand when something is happening in the treatment (or outside the treatment) that makes one or both of them want to change the plan. Understanding the function of the contact (feeling less alone, for example) can be helpful in enhancing the patient's self-understanding. Intersession contact should be used judiciously and subjects to ongoing re-evaluation to ensure its continuing utility as treatment progresses.

Answers

1. U
2. H
3. P
4. P

Principles and Clinical Pearls

1. BPD patients often seek intersession contact out of difficulty tolerating aloneness or when pushed to confront feared interpersonal situations. Clarity about expectations related to intersession contact is essential in preserving the treatment. Clinicians who are not thinking clearly about its function may inadvertently reinforce problematic dependency by being overly available or unsustainably loosening personal limits on availability in response to patients' bids for more contact.
2. The aims and frequency of intersession contact typically evolve over time when patients are progressing. The effectiveness and terms of intersession contact

should be re-evaluated and renegotiated on a regular basis with patients with respect to their progress or lack thereof. These conversations should occur during sessions and not over the phone.
3. If difficulties with intersession contact persist, a consultation is indicated to evaluate the viability of the treatment.

Case Continues...

Despite the initial difficulties, Jane faced that when exposing herself to social situations, she has been actively working with you to be more self-reliant. She makes good use of sessions to discuss underlying vulnerabilities that make these situations difficult, and to anticipate inevitable challenges before they arise. She has developed a fairly robust social life balancing time with coworkers, family, and friends. She now initiates and follows through with her own social plans. Her need for intersession contact has dramatically decreased over the last several months.

Having achieved increased stability in existing relationships, you both agree she is now in a good position to resume dating. She quickly finds a partner and feels "over the moon," astonished at her ease of connecting with this man. The relationship intensifies and she tells you of her interest in moving in with him in the fall and later marrying him. As she initiates conversations with him about the future, Jane perceives increased tension in the relationship. She is starting to feel that she wants the relationship to progress more quickly than her partner does. He tells her that he is hesitant about committing to a change in his living situation for the upcoming fall. This causes Jane to doubt the future of the relationship, and she begins regularly confronting her partner about seemingly small upsets.

You suspect that Jane's abandonment fears are prompting increased distress and reactivity within her relationship. You imagine her increasing tendency to find fault in her partner, and thereby ground to reject him, may function to protect her from being rejected by him. Despite your attempts to discuss these ideas with Jane, she denies any fear of being abandoned and instead continues to report that the relationship itself is flawed. Their fighting worsens until Jane's partner tells her that he needs a break.

After the breakup, Jane reports growing hopelessness and helplessness. She fears that this confirms her inability to have a meaningful, long-lasting relationship. She still manages to get to work but is having difficulty doing much else, including taking care of herself. She feels more depressed and suicidal, particularly on weekends when she is alone without structure or social plans but feeling tortured by negative and self-defeating thoughts. She increasingly reaches out to you between sessions during these dark times. You attempt to keep these calls short, focused, and goal oriented, but notice a pattern of her reporting increased suicidal and self-harming urges whenever you attempt to get off of the phone.

Choice Point 4

How do you handle the next call when attempts to get off of the phone during recent calls have been met by Jane reporting increased suicidal and self-harming urges?

1. Validate her understandable difficulties with loneliness and sadness about the state of her relationships, but point out that this is an opportune time to hone her capacity to manage her emotions in more independent ways that can help her to manage future inevitable distress in relationships. You emphasize the relevance of developing self-regulatory skills, briefly discuss how she intends to manage until your appointment, and then swiftly end the call (despite her stating at the end that she is afraid she may self-harm).
2. Stay on the phone, empathically validating her current difficulties, until she reports feeling more regulated and is able to commit to safety until your next session.
3. Decide to not answer this time, as you have already spoken to her several times in the last few days and believe that she has the capacity to manage until her next session.
4. Answer the phone, validate her current experience, then observe to her that her emotions escalate toward the end of each call, and express concern about this dynamic possibly promoting dependency. You validate her challenges with self-regulation but remind her that you have spoken several times in the last few days, and during that time, she has shown a capacity to manage. You express your belief that she can navigate her emotions until your next session, and remind her that you are available if she continues to struggle.

Discussion

This choice point focuses on the ways that crises can inadvertently be reinforced by the therapist during times of stress. Patients who relapse in problematic patterns following a period of stability are at risk of generating a crisis to gain desired emotional support. When these challenges emerge, therapists can inadvertently reinforce previous problematic patterns by making themselves overly available to help the patient return to baseline. Even skilled therapists struggle to be effective in these situations. Yet these scenarios present important opportunities to help patients by promoting reliance on themselves rather than on therapists. In this case, in addition to remind Jane about her own treatment goal of cultivating greater independence so that she will not "burn out" future romantic relationships, the therapist can invoke first-hand knowledge of past instances when Jane has managed herself without unboundaried intersession contact.

BPD patients can be helped by repeated psycho-education about their tendencies to overly rely on therapists to manage interpersonal losses. Therapists can enhance stability by predicting possible reversion to crisis-generating behavior to enable greater contact and support. Validating patients' inevitable pain as they learn to contend with their own and others' limitations is helpful, as is reminding them of their past capacities to manage in the face of such difficulties.

Answers

1. H
2. U
3. U
4. P

Principles and Clinical Pearls

1. BPD patients fluctuate within close relationships from being overly dependent and needy for devaluing and isolating. These shifts often occur in response to oscillating views of themselves or others as either idealized or devalued, and create instability in close relationships. Although treatment aims to help patients to integrate these extreme views into a more integrated notion of relationship, this is a lengthy process often learned through multiple exposures to relationships that swing from idealization to devaluation. In this process, providing patients with psycho-eduation about BPD-related interpersonal vulnerabilities can help them to predict and manage shifts in their view of a new partner as devalued or idealized. This can minimize the destructive impact of inevitable rifts in new romantic relationships.
2. It is helpful for therapists to anticipate a pull toward greater dependency on them when patients are at risk of losing a close relationship and become predictably more symptomatic through increased depression, anxiety, self-destructive behavior, or intersession contact. Therapists play a particularly important role during such acute struggles and can slip into becoming overly available to their patient without considering the problematic impacts this may have through reinforcing dependency on the therapist, self-destructive behavior as the most effective means of eliciting support, or patients' doubt about their own capacities to manage. Intersession contact should remain especially judicious, succinct, and goal oriented when patients are more acutely struggling.

Summary of Clinical Approach

Common challenges posed by intersession contact with BPD patients include their propensity to become overly dependent on therapists and ensuring problematic behavioral patterns that develop to maintain increased intersession support. Yet, intersession contact can help facilitate effective treatment under certain conditions, usually when parameters for its use are clearly framed at the onset of treatment and maintained thereafter. Therapists electing to be available between sessions should do so judiciously, keep contact brief and goal directed, re-evaluate over time whether intersession contact is promoting or hindering self-reliance, and predict increased dependency on such contact during times of acute difficulty. Patients benefit from having a coherent rationale for intersession contact parameters presented within psycho-education about BPD-related interpersonal vulnerabilities. Patients helped by these interventions to become more independent may still revert to problematic use of intersession contact, and therapists should maintain consistent expectations for intersession contact even during these more challenging times. At all stages of treatment, patients benefit from being reminded of the overarching treatment goal of achieving greater self-reliance and from sensing their clinicians to believe in their capacities to do so.

> **Clinician Experience: Wish to Feel Helpful by Increasing Intersession Availability**
> Many clinicians getting their initial bearings working with BPD patients feel invigorated by discovering that they can be helpful to their patients in acute crisis in between sessions. These early experiences of mastery and competence during intersession contact can feel particularly valuable for clinicians new to BPD who may otherwise feel unsure and even doubtful of their capacity to help their patients. Feeling helpful in steering someone away from acute self-harming and suicidal behavior may provide powerful reinforcement of clinicians' increased future availability.
>
> However, over time and with increasing experience, most clinicians come to better appreciate the potential long-term harms of making themselves easily available for crisis-driven intersession contact without thoroughly discussing it before, during, and after it happens. Contrary to popular belief, this is not necessary for effective BPD work. Although DBT posits that intersession contact is a key element of treatment that works, several other evidence-based treatments for BPD explicitly frame treatment around having minimal or no intersession contact. Intersession contact is, therefore, not a required common denominator in effective BPD treatment. However, as this chapter illustrates, it may be a helpful clinical tool if employed with thoughtfulness about BPD's vulnerabilities and consistency on clinicians' part.

References

1. Gunderson JG, Links P. Handbook of good psychiatric management for borderline personality disorder. Arlington: American Psychiatric Publishing, Inc; 2014.
2. Gunderson JG. Borderline patient's intolerance of aloneness: insecure attachments and therapist availability. Am J Psychiatry. 1996;153:752–8.
3. Kellogg SC, Young JE. Schema focused therapy for borderline personality disorder. J Clin Psych. 2006;62(4):445–58.
4. Linehan MM. Dialectical behavioral therapy and telephone coaching. Cog Beh Practice. 2011;18:207–8.
5. Linehan MM. DBT skills training manual. 2nd ed. New York: Guilford Publications, Inc.; 2015.
6. Jacob KL. Clinical observations about the potential benefits and pitfalls of between-session contacts with borderline patients. Harv Rev Psych. 2016;24(5):e8–14.

Dr. Jacob is the director of clinical services at the Gunderson Residence of McLean Hospital, a program specializing in the treatment of severe personality disorders with a specific focus on borderline personality disorder (BPD). She has specific training in empirically validated treatments for BPD including mentalization-based treatment, dialectical behavioral therapy, transference-focused psychotherapy, and good psychiatric management. She received her Masters and Ph.D. from Clark University and then completed her predoctoral internship at the Bedford VA followed by a postdoc at Cambridge Health Alliance. Her primary focus is on the application of empirically supported treatments for complicated clinical profiles with particular focus on BPD.

Managing Mistrust, Paranoia, and Relationship Rupture

5

Sara Rose Masland

> **Choice Point Index**
> 1. Conceptualizing patient's disclosure of past difficulties with trust
> 2. Managing worsening paranoia and feelings of disconnection
> 3. Handling patient's nonadherence to treatment and disclosure that he has an additional therapist
> 4. Responding to patient's voicemail indicating a desire to terminate treatment due to lack of trust
> 5. Deciding whether to resume care of a patient who has previously terminated treatment

Case Introduction

Alex is a 27-year-old man who was referred to you 2 weeks ago after he repeatedly canceled or no showed for individual and group dialectical behavior therapy (DBT) appointments. Both he and his previous therapist report that Alex's brief participation in DBT was not overwhelmingly helpful. Alex has a history of self-harm by burning that began in late adolescence and worsened during his participation in DBT groups. He has never been hospitalized but has been arrested as a result of impulsive behavior (e.g., drug use, reckless driving), harassment, and stalking that typically occurs during the resolution of stormy romantic relationships. He has difficulty describing his emotions and frequently expresses, "I'm just angry... just on edge, and I can't keep it down." Alex had also been issued a restraining order after stalking an ex-girlfriend in an attempt to "show her she shouldn't give up on [him]."

S. R. Masland, Ph.D.
Department of Psychology, Pomona College, Claremont, CA, USA
e-mail: sara.masland@pomona.edu

© Springer International Publishing AG, part of Springer Nature 2018
B. Palmer, B. Unruh (eds.), *Borderline Personality Disorder*,
https://doi.org/10.1007/978-3-319-90743-7_5

Alex named several barriers to effective use of DBT, including limited willingness to try DBT skills. However, his primary complaint was that he did not feel he could trust any of the other group members and believed them to be talking about him outside of group. He reported that if he spoke during group, he would leave feeling a "ball of tension" in his chest, which he attributed to his suspicion that group members were, at best, laughing at him, or, at worst, deliberately out to harm him. Alex further expressed that he has always felt like an outsider who never fits in, and that he has never told a therapist about his problems because he cannot trust anyone fully.

At this point, you have seen Alex only twice but are concerned about his ability or willingness to connect with you in a way that will facilitate effective therapy.

Choice Point 1

For each intervention, choose H: "helpful," U: "unhelpful or harmful," or P: "perhaps helpful, with reservations."

With regard to Alex's suspicion of group members and his declaration that he has never confided in his therapists due to mistrust, would you:

1. Explore whether he has complex posttraumatic stress disorder or a psychotic disorder, as either could account for his difficulty trusting others.
2. Assure him that you can be trusted.
3. Emphasize that treatment will be helpful only if you and he can find a way to collaborate.
4. Provide psycho-education about difficulties with trust in borderline personality disorder (BPD).

Discussion

It seems that Alex has been referred to you because he is not currently able to use an intensive DBT treatment owing, at least in part, to mistrust of group members and therapists alike. His level of mistrust may raise red flags about the possible presence of psychopathology other than or in addition to BPD. However, you can be reasonably sure at this point that BPD is Alex's primary diagnosis, given his pattern of stormy intimate relationships, intense efforts to avoid abandonment, impulsive behaviors, self-harm, and significant anger. Alex's paranoia can be well understood within the context of the BPD diagnosis. Although you would be wise to continue to consider other explanations, exploring other diagnoses with Alex at this point is likely to derail therapy.

However, it will likely be helpful to provide Alex with psychoeducation about the experience of paranoia or suspicion in BPD. According to the interpersonal hypersensitivity model that guides basic generalist treatment for BPD, paranoia can be explained as a symptom that results from aloneness and perceived withdrawal or rejection by others [4]. Explaining this model to Alex will help you predict together that when he is feeling suspicious of others, he will likely have more difficulty accepting help from them (and you) and may act more impulsively. Showing Alex that you are useful through psychoeducation will be more effective and genuine than simply assuring him that you are trustworthy.

After psychoeducation, the most important step you can take at this point is to outline the importance of collaboration. You should stress that for him to progress, he will need to share information about his life outside of treatment and actively collaborate with you. This mirrors the process of building healthy and stable relationships outside of therapy.

Answers

1. P
2. U
3. H
4. H

Principles and Clinical Pearls

1. Psychoeducation during the early phase of treatment has the benefit of showing the patient that you are knowledgeable and have potentially useful information. This facilitates early trust in your authority or expertise, even if more complex relational trust is absent or takes more time.
2. Significant mistrust is common in BPD and not necessarily indicative of another diagnosis. Framing mistrust/paranoia in the context of interpersonal hypersensitivity allows you and your patient to predict and plan for difficulties.
3. Collaboration between patient and therapist is essential to the success of therapy, and patients should be made aware early that they are expected to be active partners in the process of change.

Case Continues...

Over the next few weeks, Alex seems receptive to psychoeducation and appreciative of learning more about BPD. He seems to be collaborating with you and reports that he is beginning to trust you. However, Alex soon misses an appointment without notifying you in advance. When he next returns, he explains that he broke up with a girlfriend he had been seeing for 2 months and then had a verbal and physical altercation with a good friend. Since these incidents, he has been isolating alone at home, feeling "disconnected from everything." He has begun to believe that his girlfriend must have left him for his friend, despite the fact that they had never met. He also expresses the belief that if he tells you the full extent of his dysregulation after the breakup, you will "betray" him by ending treatment.

Choice Point 2

With regard to Alex's worsening paranoia and disconnection, would you:

1. Begin an antipsychotic medication.
2. Reassure Alex that his paranoia is the result of cognitive distortions, not reality.
3. Suggest that Alex finds a way to structure his day with meaningful activity, preferably work.
4. Explicitly link Alex's feelings of increased mistrust to recent interpersonal conflicts.
5. Explain to Alex that his paranoia is likely the manifestation of an underlying fantasy that involves being controlled, manipulated, or used in a degrading manner.

Discussion

The number of randomized controlled trials examining pharmacotherapy for BPD is limited to approximately 33 [12]. No medication has proven consistently or considerably helpful, and none has been approved by the FDA for treating BPD. However, antipsychotics may be useful for cognitive or perceptual BPD symptoms, such as transient stress-induced paranoia, perceptual disturbances, or dissociation [5]. Antipsychotics may also decrease anger and impulse control [9, 14]. Their use for any reason in BPD should be frequently reassessed and ideally tapered or discontinued over time after stability is achieved, as patients with BPD are commonly subject to high levels of psychotropic polypharmacy [10, 15]. Pro re nata (PRN; as needed) use of antipsychotics for agitation is common but should be minimized, as high levels of PRN medication use are associated with unrecovered BPD patients [7]. Existing guidelines and clinical wisdom highlight the importance of enlisting patients' collaboration in initiating, monitoring, and tapering all categories of psychotropic medications to avoid common iatrogenic harms [11].

Reassurance that Alex need not be so paranoid or suspicious is likely to be perceived as invalidating at this point. However, invoking the interpersonal hypersensitivity model could help Alex understand why he might be more prone to paranoid or distrustful thought patterns following the dissolution of his relationship and conflict with his friend. This may also be a good opportunity to highlight that romantic relationships are often destabilizing for patients with BPD, and that building structure, routine, and purpose through employment will provide Alex with an impetus for continued social contact (rather than isolation) and social rehabilitation.

Finally, deep interpretation of Alex's paranoia, however, accurate or insightful, is likely to be perceived as intrusive (possibly exacerbating his paranoia) and unlikely to facilitate change.

Answers

1. P
2. P
3. H
4. H
5. U

Principles and Clinical Pearls

1. Chaotic interpersonal relationships can destabilize patients' experience of themselves and the world, causing or exacerbating cognitive-perceptual symptoms of paranoia, mistrust, and dissociation. Clinicians should actively use the interpersonal hypersensitivity model of BPD to explore with patients within a psychoeducational framework whether these symptoms relate to recent interpersonal experiences.
2. Basic generalist management of BPD stresses the importance of helping patients achieve "work before love," as achieving productive employment and meaningful activity is more likely to stabilize trust and prosocial behavior than serial, tumultuous romantic relationships.
3. Antipsychotic medications have an adjunctive role in the management of BPD-related mistrust and paranoia. Patients should be enlisted to collaborate in monitoring their usefulness and potential harmful effects.

Case Continues…

Alex again responds well to your efforts at psychoeducation and agrees to try an antipsychotic medication. He ultimately discloses the extent of his impulsivity following the breakup and expresses relief and appreciation that you do not terminate treatment as a result. Treatment continues, and you seem to be building an alliance. However, within a few weeks, Alex reports that he has started to see another clinician and that he has not been taking his antipsychotic medication. He reports that your efforts to encourage him to find employment have made him feel "worthless and invalidated," and that he feels you "pry too much for information."

Choice Point 3

How would you respond to Alex's disclosure that he has started to see another therapist and has not been taking medications as prescribed?

1. Interpret this as an aggressive act against you.
2. Ask Alex directly if he remembers your conversation about the need to follow prescription guidelines and collaborate in monitoring medication usefulness.
3. Have a frank discussion with Alex about whether treatment has been useful, and if it would make clinical sense for him to switch providers.
4. "Lean out": step back from asking for information about Alex's life outside of treatment, so that he does not perceive you as intrusive and even harder to trust.
5. Apologize for any way you might have contributed to Alex's feeling of invalidation but stand by and review your rationale for why finding employment is essential for optimal recovery.

Discussion

Alex has now ruptured cooperation by initiating therapy with another provider and failing to follow prescription guidelines. Your response should be active but not reactive. Interpreting Alex's behavior as an aggressive act against you may have some validity but may also be perceived as reactive and is unlikely to be clinically useful. This is a time to be thoughtful and to hold the patient accountable for remembering and using treatment without becoming reactive. This is achieved by asking Alex directly about what he made of your recommendations concerning following prescription guidelines and collaborating with you, and why he has not implemented them.

Now is another good time to reemphasize for Alex that he must be an active participant in evaluating whether treatment is working. You have some reason to believe treatment may not be helping, as Alex is not following your instructions. Alternatively, Alex may have sought another provider as an "attachment bid" to gain support from you through eliciting your caring, concerned response. Regardless of your hypothesis about why Alex seems to have discarded your recommendations, now is a time to discuss whether treatment should continue.

A common and understandable for clinicians to have when patients become mistrustful is to step back or "lean out." Often clinicians fear that further questioning or expressions of concern may be perceived as intrusive for wary patients. However, patients benefit when clinicians "lean into" the interaction by taking an active stance around helping them to understand that this type of behavior ruptures cooperation and may indicate a need for changes in the treatment. It can help to explain the bind you are in as a clinician when a patient requests that you act in a counterproductive manner: "I understand that when I ask questions I may seem like I am trying to get information, and that is true. But I believe I would be doing you a disservice by not asking about your life outside of treatment."

"Leaning in" also involves recognizing the difficulties that we create for patients in pressing treatment goals they often do not initially embrace of their own accord. It is easy to bungle the delivery of a requirement for employment in a way that leaves patients feeling criticized or misunderstood, but we can manage this by apologizing for any mistakes we have made along the way in lack of sensitivity or empathy for their plight, reiterating clear rationales for our recommendations, and conveying genuine interest and curiosity about patients' responses to what we say. Most patients with BPD come to eventually understand why you so firmly recommend, and even require, employment.

Answers

1. U
2. H
3. P
4. U
5. H

Principles and Clinical Pearls

1. Be active, not reactive, in discussing relationship ruptures and noncompliance with treatment recommendations. "Lean into" the discussion thoughtfully and humbly, but without backing away from sound evidence-based recommendations.
2. Hold patients accountable for remembering and making use of previous discussions.
3. Emphasize that treatment should continue "so long as it is useful," and that patients are expected to collaborate in monitoring treatment effectiveness.

Case Continues...

Alex reacts negatively to your wish to discuss whether treatment is working, but eventually joins in the conversation. He leaves your office reporting that he intends to cancel with the other therapist and continue with you. However, he leaves you a voicemail message a few days later stating: "I'm done with treatment. I don't trust that you are really on my side. If you were, you wouldn't push me so much to get a job and talk about my life. I cancelled with the other therapist, too. I'm just going to take care of myself from now on."

Choice Point 4

How would you respond to Alex's message?

1. Call back, express concern, and insist that Alex continue to see you.
2. Call back and, if you cannot reach him, take measures to ensure he is not at imminent risk of serious self-harm (e.g., by asking police to perform a safety check or issuing an order for involuntary evaluation for hospitalization).

3. Do not return Alex's call, as he has made it clear that he is done with you.
4. Call back, express concern, and offer a referral to another provider or treatment or a meeting with you to discuss his concerns.

Discussion

Treatment should continue only "so long as it is helpful." At this point, Alex seems unready to use treatment to change in the are as you deem most crucial. Insisting that Alex continue to see you without evidence that it is useful sets you both up for continued frustration and may create or reinforce the notion that treatment should continue supportively without expectation of change. On the other hand, not calling back at all may be considered negligent. You should return the call, but if he does not respond, aggressively trying to ensure his safety seems unwarranted because he has not made any expressions of intent to harm himself and does not have a history of suicide attempts.

The best course of action is to call Alex back, express your concern, and offer an appropriate treatment referral according to a recently proposed stepped model of BPD treatment [1]. In this model, patients with early or low-severity problems and those who have not benefitted from more intensive evidence-based treatments are those best routed to lower intensity treatment approaches. Alex has longstanding, somewhat severe problems, and has not benefited from your generalist approach or from a past trial of DBT. Referral to another specialty evidence-based treatment may perpetuate his unproductive engagement with treatment. Most prudent would be a referral to another generalist clinician or case manager who will pare down the intensity of treatment to match a projected slower pace of change.

Answers

1. U
2. U
3. U
4. H

Principles and Clinical Pearls

1. Treatment should continue only if it is useful. Change is expected.
2. At the time of termination, the referrals you offer should reflect your assessment of the degree of change achieved (or not) during your treatment and of their likelihood to change with more, less, or similarly intensive treatment approaches.

Case Continues...

You leave a message for Alex expressing your concern about his choice to end all treatment abruptly. You also offer a referral to a lower intensity treatment you imagine might be easier for him to tolerate. You do not hear from him for 6 months, at which point he calls and asks to restart treatment with you. He explains that when he terminated treatment, he was actually starting to trust you, which scared him. He also reports that he has started working part time at a pet supply store and has found this very helpful.

Choice Point 5

How would you respond to Alex's request to see you again?

1. Refuse, noting that treatment did not work before so is unlikely to be helpful now.
2. Refuse, and once again refer him to another clinician.
3. Praise his progress by saying, "I knew a job would help you! I'm so proud of you!"
4. Agree to see him again and pick up where you left off.
5. Agree to see him again, being very careful to emphasize the need for collaboration and the expectation for change.

Discussion

Refusal to help connect Alex to treatment in any way would be negligent. However, you must evaluate your own willingness and ability to work with Alex again. You may have experienced some burnout or compassion fatigue if the treatment felt difficult for you to stick with in the past, and this would be a good reason for you to suggest another treater could be more useful to him now. Should you re-engage, Alex's wish to re-initiate treatment, his admission that he was beginning to trust you, and his follow-through on finding employment all bode well. If you choose to see Alex again, it is more important to set firm expectations for change and collaboration than to offer effusive encouragements that may be perceived as cloying. It is more useful to validate Alex's progress and encourage it to continue.

Answers

1. U
2. P

3. U
4. U
5. H

Principles and Clinical Pearls

1. For clients prone to paranoid ideas and general mistrust, the road to building an alliance may be long and rocky.
2. Treatment breaks provide an opportunity to re-establish and re-affirm a change-oriented treatment frame.

Summary of Clinical Approach

Therapeutic alliance is an important mediator of treatment effectiveness across disorders. Yet patients with BPD have specific difficulties with forming stable, trusting bonds, and may experience significant suspiciousness or paranoia, particularly during times of stress. In this context, establishing a trusting relationship can feel like a fast-moving target for both clinicians and patients. Conceptualizing the symptom of paranoia within the the framework of interpersonal hypersensitivity is helpful for delivering effective psychoeducation to patients, and for maintaining compassion and mitigating burnout for clinicians. Clinicians working with individuals who have difficulty with interpersonal trust should provide psychoeducation early, be clear about expectations for active collaboration, and be active but not reactive when alliance is ruptured. The expectation for change should not be lost in the struggle to form a trusting relationship, and clinicians must be reflective about whether treatment is helping and should continue (or begin again, in the case of termination). In addition, prescribers should be cautious and judicious about the use of antipsychotic medications.

Clinician Experience: Expecting and Managing Difficulties with Trust and Cooperation

A strong body of research now confirms the clinical impression that people with BPD view others as untrustworthy and behave accordingly. They have a response bias to rate others as untrustworthy [3], particularly in the context of negative emotion [8]. In behavioral exchange paradigms, or "trust games," requiring individuals to cooperate with others to reap maximum financial benefit, people with BPD have lower hopes that their partners will act in a trustworthy manner, are themselves less cooperative, and are more likely to rupture cooperation [6, 13]. These findings support the common clinical experience that building trust with patients with BPD can be difficult, and it should not be wholly unexpected (or personalized) when patients rupture cooperation, as in Alex's case.

In addition, individuals with BPD process violations of social expectations differently than healthy populations at the levels of neural processing and self-report. They expect extreme inclusion from relationship partners and are likely to perceive rejection even when included "fairly" in group interactions [2]. This means that even when you feel active and engaged in a treatment, your patient may readily perceive rejection or disconnection from you, hindering normal relational processes that facilitate trust. On a neural level, when trust is ruptured by another party, people with BPD show patterns of activity distinct from those in healthy controls [6]. Familiarizing yourself with these studies both informs your appreciation for your patient's struggles to build a trusting alliance and equips you with psychoeducational concepts useful for helping patients understand why they so often feel left out, rejected, and betrayed—experiences they may have at times with you.

References

1. Choi-Kain LW, Albert EB, Gunderson JG. Evidence-based treatments for borderline personality disorder: Implementation, integration, and stepped care. Harvard Rev Psychiatry. 2016;24(5):342–56.
2. De Panfilis C, Riva P, Preti E, Cabrino C, Marchesi C. When social inclusion is not enough: implicit expectations of extreme inclusion in borderline personality disorder. Personal Disord. 2015;6(4):301–9.
3. Fertuck EA, Grinband J, Stanley B. Facial trust appraisal negatively biased in borderline personality disorder. Psychiatry Res. 2013;207(3):195–202.
4. Gunderson JG, Links PS. Handbook of good psychiatric management for borderline personality disorder: American Psychiatric Pub; Washington, D.C., USA. 2014.
5. Ingenhoven TJ, Duivenvoorden HJ. Differential effectiveness of antipsychotics in borderline personality disorder: meta-analyses of placebo-controlled, randomized clinical trials on symptomatic outcome domains. J Clin Psychopharmacol. 2011;31(4):489–96.
6. King-Casas B, Sharp C, Lomax-Bream L, Lohrenz T, Fonagy P, Montague PR. The rupture and repair of cooperation in borderline personality disorder. Science. 2008;321(5890):806–10.
7. Martinho E Jr, Fitzmaurice GM, Frankenburg FR, Zanarini MC. Pro re nata (as needed) psychotropic medication use in patients with borderline personality disorder and subjects with other personality disorders over 14 years of prospective follow-up. J Clin Psychopharmacol. 2014;34(4):499–503.
8. Masland, SR, Hooley, JM. When trust does not come easily: Negative emotional information unduly influences trust judgments for individuals with borderline personality traits. (unpublished manuscript).
9. Mercer D, Douglass AB, Links PS. Meta-analysis of mood-stabilizers, antidepressants and antipsychotics in the treatment of borderline personality disorder: effectiveness for depression and anger symptoms. J Personal Disord. 2009;23:156–74.

10. Paolini E, Mezzetti FA, Pierri F, Moretti P. Pharmacological treatment of borderline personality disorder: a retrospective observational study at inpatient unit in Italy. Int J Psychiatry Clin Pract. 2017;21(1):75–9.
11. Silk KR. The process of managing medications in patients with borderline personality disorder. J Psychiatr Pract. 2011;17(5):311–9.
12. Stoffers JM, Lieb K. Pharmacotherapy for borderline personality disorder – current evidence and recent trends. Curr Psychiatry Rep. 2015;17:534.
13. Unoka Z, Seres I, Áspán N, Bódi N, Kéri S. Trust game reveals restricted interpersonal transactions in patients with borderline personality disorder. J Personal Disord. 2009;23(4):399–409.
14. Vita A, De Peri L, Sacchetti E. Antipsychotics, antidepressants, anticonvulsants, and placebo on the syptom dimensions of borderline personality disorder: a meta-analysis of randomized controlled and open-label trials. J Clin Psychopharmacol. 2011;31(5):613–24.
15. Zanarini MC, Frankenburg FR, Harned A, Fitzmaurice G. Rates of psychotropic medication use reported by borderline patients and axis II comparison subjects over 16 years of prospective follow-up. J Clin Psychopharmacol. 2015;35(1):63–7.

Dr. Masland is an Assistant Professor of Psychology at Pomona College. She is a graduate of the clinical psychology doctoral program at Harvard University and completed her post-doctoral clinical research fellowship at McLean Hospital, where she worked primarily at the Gunderson Residence, an intensive residential treatment program for women with severe personality disorders. She maintains an active research laboratory dedicated to understanding and attenuating stigma about borderline personality disorder and to clarifying deficits in social cognition (e.g., stress-related transient paranoia) associated with the disorder.

Emergency Department Management

6

Victor Hong and Steven Bartek

Choice Point Index
1. Principles for organizing an interview in the ED
2. Clarifying experience rather than reacting to behaviors
3. Focusing on events leading to the emergency department visit
4. Managing anger and empathic failures
5. Prioritizing treatment interventions in a straightforward manner

Case Introduction

Frank is a 24-year-old graduate student who is seen in the emergency department following an overdose. He reportedly took 7 pills of acetaminophen and 5 pills of diphenhydramine. He had been drinking and is intoxicated. His drug screen is positive for cannabis. He was brought to the emergency department after he posted on social media that he was "done with life," prompting a 9-1-1 call by his friend. He is medically cleared by the emergency physician and you are then consulted to assess his safety risk. The emergency department staff indicates that he has been "gamey" and that he "won't talk." A nurse says "good luck" as you enter his room. He is in treatment with an outpatient therapist, and his primary care doctor has been prescribing him sertraline and alprazolam for "depression and anxiety." He has presented to the emergency department in the past for intoxication and cutting behaviors. When you enter the room, Frank's eyes are downcast, he is texting furiously on his phone, and he looks irritable.

V. Hong, M.D. · S. Bartek, M.D. (✉)
Department of Psychiatry, University of Michigan, Ann Arbor, MI, USA
e-mail: sbartek@med.umich.edu

© Springer International Publishing AG, part of Springer Nature 2018
B. Palmer, B. Unruh (eds.), *Borderline Personality Disorder*,
https://doi.org/10.1007/978-3-319-90743-7_6

Choice Point 1

For each choice point, choose H: "helpful," U: "unhelpful or harmful," or P: "perhaps helpful, with reservations."

After introducing yourself, you:

1. Express concern about Frank and how he is doing.
2. Explain that most people who take overdoses require a psychiatric hospitalization and that will be the focus of your discussion.
3. Keep your distance, as you do not want to be in an unsafe situation with a potentially agitated patient.
4. Ask Frank to explain what brought him to the emergency department.
5. Inquire about who he was texting.

Discussion

Managing patients with BPD in an emergency setting, such as a medical or psychiatric ED, requires a unique set of skills and a heightened attention to detail, as you are often dealing with acute suicidality and agitation in patients who are, by definition, in crisis. Often, evaluations need to be handled expeditiously, and dispositions can be challenging. BPD patients frequently present to EDs and do so recurrently. Their presence can add a chaotic element to an already tumultuous backdrop [1]. When managing patients with BPD in the ED, a practical and organized approach is crucial [2]. Especially challenging aspects of care can include responding to self-harm and suicidal behavior [3], managing disruptive activity, and coping with the staff's and one's own countertransference reactions [4].

As with any patient in crisis, but particularly those with the interpersonal hypersensitivity inherent in most patients with BPD, your initial approach is critical to developing rapport and a therapeutic alliance. Patients with BPD can be extraordinarily keyed into their interactions with others and may require repeated validation of their pain and suffering. Opening your interview with statements expressing genuine concern may serve to portray you as someone who wants to help and who is unlikely to reject the patient.

One of the primary pitfalls in responding to BPD patients in crisis is jumping to the conclusion that every attempt to harm themselves necessitates an inpatient hospitalization. This clinician response is frequently due to excessive anxiety regarding liability risk. Although inpatient care is indeed indicated for those whose acute suicidal risk is high, often self-injurious behavior is not reflective of suicidal urges. Thus, it is important to carefully assess the dangerousness of the situation before introducing the idea of hospitalization to the patient.

Certainly, with a truly agitated patient, it is important to consider your own safety. But in the absence of any clear indicators of violence risk, keeping your distance or being dismissive of a BPD patient will likely prompt a negative reaction, cause them to shut down, and preclude a meaningful exchange.

Engaging the patient in problem solving is helpful in the emergency setting, as patients themselves, when supported, may identify the best solutions to their predicament. However, BPD patients may be hesitant to open up. If met with passivity, you can explain that your ability to help them depends on their participation in the dialog and decision making.

It may be helpful to know more about the interpersonal world of the patient. In this case, knowing who Frank is texting may give you clues into the cause and details of his crisis and may potentially help you identify individuals in his sphere of social support to assist in safety planning. That being said, it is worth balancing this with not being unnecessarily intrusive early in the interaction.

Answers

1. H
2. U
3. U
4. H
5. P

Principles and Clinical Pearls

1. To increase the potential of a safe disposition from the emergency department, approach a patient with possible BPD in an engaged, genuinely concerned fashion.
2. Do not overreact to a patient's suicidal or self-injurious behavior. Pay close attention and engage in a measured discussion about true suicidal risk and what interpersonal factors may be contributing to the crisis at hand.

Case Continues...

You ask Frank what led to his overdose today, and he says "I don't know," barely looking up. You explain that you want to help, but to do so you need his assistance. After all, you tell him, you are not a very good "mind reader." Following an awkward pause, he says, "No one cares so what's the point?" You encourage him to tell you more, and he explains that he has been struggling with a relationship. His girlfriend has seemed distant recently and has openly questioned if she wants the relationship to continue. Frank says this has caused his mood to be "all over the place." You say that the relationship sounds stressful. He notes that since he arrived at the ED, multiple friends and family members, including his girlfriend, have sent him messages of support.

Choice Point 2

At this point in the interview, you say:

1. "I know how you feel; I've been through a similar thing with my partner."
2. "Do you think that your relationship stress led to your overdose attempt?"
3. "What's it like to receive all that support from loved ones?"
4. "It's important that we know whether you were actually trying to kill yourself; we don't want to take any risks."

Discussion

Measured self-disclosure can be helpful in demonstrating to a patient that you understand their plight. The clinical relationship, while brief and professional, is real, with genuine emotions and reactions to each other. However, disclosing specifics about your life and relationship history should be avoided and is likely to engender a sense that your relationship with the patient is more personal than professional. With this boundary in mind, replying with an authentic display of empathy is certainly recommended and can enhance the patient's trust in you, a caring provider.

If the patient does not readily make the (likely) connection between his interpersonal stressors and his overdose attempt, explicitly underscoring the potential association can help, especially if you suspect he has BPD. The sooner he understands the role of relationship stressors in his problems, the better, as managing his sensitivity to feeling unsupported and preoccupied with others can then become a target of his treatment.

It is valuable to understand the BPD patient in the context of their social supports, or lack thereof. How Frank reacts to increased levels of support from his social circle can illuminate aspects of his character traits and may also inform how likely it is that you will reach a reasonable safety plan that facilitates discharge from the ED without hospitalization.

Ultimately it will be necessary to determine Frank's intent in taking an overdose of pills. A comprehensive suicide risk assessment is required, and it is important to document your assessment. However, be mindful that if the BPD patient perceives that you are focused more on reducing liability than on their well-being, then the therapeutic alliance will suffer. Without a sufficient alliance, navigating the interview, and planning the ultimate disposition of the patient, will be challenging tasks. Constructing a shared understanding of his suicidal narrative is consistent with effective risk assessment.

Answers

1. U
2. H
3. H
4. U

Principles and Clinical Pearls

1. Interpersonal hypersensitivity is at the core of borderline personality disorder. When working with a patient who exhibits multiple BPD traits, search for a possible interpersonal trigger for a patient's suicidal or self-harming behavior. You may quickly unearth why they are presenting to the emergency department and the root cause of the present crisis.
2. Strive to learn about the patient's social supports and how he reacts to others, both positively and negatively. These data will help you shape an appropriate disposition.

Case Continues...

Frank says he was not thinking about what he was doing when he took the overdose, admitting he was drunk. He tells you that it feels good to get support from his friends and family but doubts the support is genuine, saying, "I have trust issues." You respond that this sounds important to explore further. You learn he frequently has conflicts with friends and family, which then causes him to feel "panicky" and become acutely depressed. He has coped by cutting himself superficially since he was 16 years old. He has previously taken overdoses, all of which he describes as impulsive and happening when he felt "out of control." He qualifies this further by saying "I don't even know if most of them were real suicide attempts, I just didn't want to feel terrible anymore."

Choice Point 3

At this point in the interview, you:

1. Inform him that he has borderline personality disorder.
2. Ask him to discuss events leading up to his overdose in detail, and complete a preliminary "chain analysis."
3. Tell him that he will need to sign a "safety contract" saying he will not kill himself to be discharged from the emergency department.
4. Suggest that if he becomes this upset with his girlfriend, it is likely an unhealthy relationship that should end.
5. Mention his alcohol and marijuana use and how it may have contributed to the overdose.

Discussion

Psycho-education is essential to effectively manage patients with BPD. Good psycho-education can debunk myths about BPD, help patients to better understand their patterns of behaviors and emotions, and may help set realistic expectations of the prognosis and treatment options. In this case, Frank demonstrates many symptoms consistent with BPD, rather than classic depression and anxiety. Although it may sometimes be premature to formally diagnosis BPD after a single assessment in an emergency setting, when clear signs are present, it is important to unapologetically offer your professional opinion about BPD's likely role in the patient's distress. In this case and most others involving BPD, the connection between relationship sensitivity and his impulsive behaviors is important to point out.

Frank has suggested that previous episodes of cutting and suicide attempts have occurred when he was acutely distressed, but he has not shared a narrative for the recent overdose. By closely exploring the events leading up to his overdose, you can help illuminate precipitating factors. Equipped with a better understanding of crisis triggers, the patient may have more opportunities for utilizing coping techniques, earlier intervention in the future, and more effective and meaningful safety planning.

Safety contracts, while sometimes used in practice, have limited evidence for decreasing risk of future suicide attempts and offer no medicolegal protection. The presence of a safety contract, if used at all, should not prevent a clinician from completing a thorough safety risk assessment. However, working with the patient, family, and any outpatient providers to develop a safety plan - including signs of impending crisis, potential coping strategies, who to contact, and how to maintain a safe environment - can give the patient a concrete strategy for the future.

At this point, not enough is known about the nature of the patient's relationship to say if it is healthy or unhealthy. Recommending the termination (or continuation) of a relationship falls outside of the ED clinician's role, and approaching his relationship in this way would likely encourage the patient to avoid examining his role in the conflict.

Substance use disorders are frequently comorbid with BPD, and disinhibition from substances can increase the patient's risk of attempting and completing suicide. It is an important topic to bring up in this setting, as part of further psychoeducation, particularly when discussing safety planning.

Answers

1. P
2. H
3. U
4. U
5. H

Principles and Clinical Pearls

1. An open discussion about a possible BPD diagnosis, along with written materials, can help explain a patient's behavior, assist the patient in focusing expectations, and inform them of the treatment options that are likely to be most helpful.

2. Perform a "chain analysis" and examine events that may have led to a BPD patient's crisis. This can help them identify triggers, likely interpersonal in nature, and the findings can then be included in a safety plan.
3. Substance use disorders commonly co-occur with BPD and should be identified, discussed with the patient, and factored into the safety assessment.

Case Continues...

Frank says he does not know about "the borderline thing," but he will look into it. As you work through a "chain analysis" with him, it becomes apparent that his overdose was preceded by his girlfriend telling him she would not go on a trip with him as planned, but would instead spend the time with her friends. He realizes this irritated him greatly. Moments later Frank becomes distracted by a text message. He curses loudly and says, "She's impossible! I wish I had really killed myself!" Responding to the commotion, a staff member steps into the room to check in, then leaves after you reassure them that all is fine. Frank says, "Everyone's mad at me now. I'm done!" You are caught off guard by his sudden outburst and feel your heart begin to race.

Choice Point 4

In response to Frank's outburst, you say:

1. "Would you like some medication to help calm down?"
2. "I always like to get other points of view. Is there someone I could talk to about you?"
3. "You seem very upset. Can you help me understand why?"
4. "I'm concerned about your safety, especially when you talk about killing yourself. Let's talk about that."
5. "You cannot shout and speak like that here!" You raise your voice somewhat to get your point across.

Discussion

Medication can indeed be useful in calming a patient if they are either so distressed they cannot engage in an assessment or are an imminent threat to themselves or others. However, in this case, there is no indication that verbal de-escalation would be ineffective, and quickly offering medications to Frank reinforces the notion that medications are the best solution to the problem of his excessive anger.

Reaching out for collateral information is an essential component of the safety assessment in an emergency setting, particularly for patients with BPD, given the added weight that their relationships carry. Attempts should be made to contact outpatient providers, and friends or family members who can provide valuable information regarding recent events and help with safety planning. That said, it would be important to address the patient's intense affect before making this request, as he may reject the notion of contacting others about him in a moment of anger. Even if the patient ultimately refuses to allow contact with people in his life, it is nonetheless a necessary step if safety is in question.

When BPD patients are distressed, identifying and addressing affect can help them de-escalate and demonstrate you are paying attention. Here, this would be another opportunity for Frank to actively participate in exploring his reaction, potentially helping him better understand the connection between his relationship stress and his emotions and behaviors.

With his comment, "I wish I had really killed myself," Frank has provided you an entree into an open discussion about his safety. This topic should be approached, as always, with genuine concern, and with a focus on any acute risk factors above and beyond what you understand to be Frank's static risk factors. Pay close attention to countertransference to avoid initiating unnecessary hospitalization due to provider anxiety, or conversely, conducting an inadequate safety assessment due to frustration and hopelessness.

While emotional dysregulation is common in BPD patients in crisis, providers must take care not to become dysregulated themselves in responding to them. It may require considerable focus and intention to keep calm and communicate with distressed patients in a professional manner.

Answers

1. U
2. P
3. H
4. H
5. U

Principles and Clinical Pearls

1. Individuals with BPD can present with intense emotional reactivity, which providers should attempt to address with verbal de-escalation rather than with medication [5]. For BPD patients, medications should be viewed as adjunctive, with psychotherapy and other psychosocial interventions as the core modalities of treatment. Giving patients the impression that medications are the answer for mood lability will reinforce inappropriate expectations regarding their efficacy.
2. When treating BPD patients in the ED, communicating with collateral informants is crucial to conduct the safety assessment and to formulate a good dis-

position plan. It also reduces liability risk by ensuring that you have all necessary information about possible risk factors, have evaluated the adequacy of the outpatient treatment, and understand the level of available social support.
3. It is important to consider the BPD patient's safety in the context of acute-on-chronic risk whereby you accept that at baseline, patients with BPD have an elevated chronic risk of suicide which should rarely guide the decision to hospitalize or not. To reach an appropriate and safe disposition, providers should focus primarily on acute stressors and risk factors (see sidebar). Clinicians must recognize and manage any excessive countertransference so as to engage in a sober and comprehensive discussion regarding safety.

The Case Continues...

Frank shares that his girlfriend texted that she is worried about him but is upset that, once again, he has ruined her plans by "losing it." He feels that as his alprazolam dose was decreased, he has "definitely been more on edge," and he asks you to prescribe a higher dose. With some pressing from you, he tells you he often says things he does not mean, including that he should kill himself. He actually wants to live and mentions that he looks forward to his career after graduate school, has family members that would be devastated if he killed himself, and enjoys sports. He tells you when people anger him, he lashes out before he thinks about what to say. After some time venting about his problems, he seems calmer. He says, "Just give me my prescription and let me go home. Nothing is going to really help in the long run, but I might as well try that."

Choice Point 5

With this new information, you:

1. Ask whom among his social supports can be contacted to collaborate with him in developing a safe discharge plan.
2. Tell him to stay away from his girlfriend, as she clearly agitates him and should be avoided given "the heat of the moment."
3. Respond to his requests for benzodiazepines by expressing concern that he is addicted to alprazolam.
4. Provide information about the prognosis for people with BPD, and the likelihood that, over time, he will get better.
5. Reiterate that it appears his relationship difficulties significantly impact him, and that moving forward, his sensitivity in relationships should be a focus of treatment.

Discussion

If discharge to home is the likely disposition, then it is imperative to include the BPD patient's social supports and outpatient providers in the plan. They can assist by supporting patients in participating in close follow-up care, distracting them from interpersonal stressors, and ensuring that they feel cared for and supported. All of the above will enhance the safety of the discharge plan, and ideally the patient is enlisted to help generate some of these plans.

It is not reasonable to expect Frank to avoid contact with his girlfriend, even if doing so could be helpful in the short term. A more beneficial strategy may be to discuss ways in which Frank can manage specific issues in the relationship that may be particularly upsetting. Role playing can be an important tool here.

Navigating the issue of medications with BPD patients can be challenging, as they frequently insist that medication changes are what is needed in times of crisis. However, medications have not been proven to be significantly or consistently helpful to treat core BPD symptoms, and relying on them is a setup for disappointment [6]. Benzodiazepines in particular should be avoided whenever possible given they can disinhibit patients, and when taken with other sedating medications, they can be dangerous in overdose. Benzodiazepine use is made more problematic by the fact that substance use is a common comorbidity with BPD. However, confronting a BPD patient about medication dependence or misuse is likely to induce defensiveness. Good psycho-education about the evidence for medication risks and rewards is likely to be less provocative and more effective.

Engendering a sense of hope, even in the midst of a crisis is an important step to take. For the vast majority of those with BPD, symptoms will remit over time. Providers can validate the intense hopelessness BPD patients feel while, at the same time, providing a confident professional endorsement of hope for their improvement.

Highlighting that interpersonal hypersensitivity significantly impacts Frank's symptoms and behaviors is a helpful intervention to repeat throughout the clinical interaction in order to increase his awareness of core problems [7]. When BPD patients explore this fundamental connection, over time they will better understand themselves and gain insight into how to cope with crises.

Answers

1. H
2. P
3. U
4. H
5. H

Principles and Clinical Pearls

1. Significant medication changes should not be made in times of crisis despite a BPD patient's insistence. If any medication changes are implemented, they should be done so only with the participation of the patient's outpatient providers.

2. Communication is a key in an emergency setting, particularly when safety is in question.
3. Good psycho-education regarding core aspects of BPD including interpersonal hypersensitivity and likely prognosis is critical.

The Case Continues…

Frank's family and a good friend are contacted, but the ED staff is unable to reach the outpatient providers. His family agrees to be active in supporting him in coming days and his friend arrives to the ED and plans on staying with him upon discharge. After hearing these plans, Frank's affect becomes notably brighter. You determine that despite his self-injurious behavior and ingestion of pills, there was no true suicidal intent, and therefore, discharge is reasonably safe. The patient and his family say that they are committed to contacting his therapist and primary care doctor and will also set up an appointment with a psychiatrist. You provide him with referrals to psychiatrists in the area and schedule a follow-up phone call to assess his progress and outpatient care plans. Although you feel somewhat concerned about discharging Frank, you are comforted by how he is responding to the considerable support he is receiving.

Summary of Clinical Approach

When clinicians encounter BPD patients in the ED setting challenges may include managing acute self-injurious and suicidal behavior, intoxication, anger, interpersonal hypersensitivity, diagnostic confusion, and requests for medication changes. It is imperative to approach the BPD patient in an active, genuinely concerned manner while keeping one's emotional reactions in check. Attempts to determine likely interpersonal stressors may help the provider expeditiously locate the trigger point for the crisis and can improve the safety risk assessment, which must be done in a grounded, organized way, guided by the principle of acute-on-chronic risk. Psycho-education about the probable role of BPD can assist the patient in understanding their reactions and can provide the patient a useful framework regarding which interventions are likely to be helpful (psychosocial) or not (medications). Communication with colleagues, the patient's social supports, and their outpatient providers is paramount in reaching the most appropriate disposition.

Clinician Experience: Acute-On-Chronic Risk
A useful but not always well-understood concept in assessing suicide risk in BPD patients is the acute-on-chronic risk model. BPD patients have a higher chronic risk of suicide when compared with the general population, and clinicians can become highly anxious when assessing these patients in crisis. However, chronic risk factors are not generally modifiable in an inpatient setting and, therefore, should not drive the decision of whether or not to

hospitalize a BPD patient. Relying too heavily on chronic risk factors in clinical decision making can lead to unnecessary inpatient admissions, which, if recurrent, can foster dependency in patients and interfere with long-term improvement. Patients who persistently seek hospitalization due to their chronic symptoms can be educated that good outpatient treatment and psychosocial interventions are likely to be more effective to help manage chronic issues than an inpatient stay. All of these considerations should be documented in the medical record. Acute risk factors in BPD patients include worsening depression, concurrent substance abuse, recent discharge from a hospital, loss or perceived loss of support, and presenting in a regressed state. Clinicians must assess for these issues along with considering other elements of a comprehensive safety assessment, such as intent and plan for suicide and access to means. If acute risk factors are present, attempts should be made to reduce such risks in the ED setting and consider inpatient hospitalization if they persist. Inadequate safety assessments can be another dangerous pitfall when considering acute versus chronic risk factors. If clinicians are too focused on the chronicity of the BPD patients' symptoms, (e.g., that the patient is always suicidal, so there is no point to hospitalizing them), then they may overlook acute risk factors. Such oversight can increase liability, compromise sound decision making, and may lead to adverse events.

References

1. Boggild AK, Heisel MJ, Links PS. Social, demographic, and clinical factors related to disruptive behaviour in hospital. Can J Psychiatr. 2004;49:114–8.
2. Hong V. Borderline personality disorder in the emergency department: good psychiatric management. Harv Rev Psychiatry. 2016;24(5):357–66.
3. Zaheer J, Links PS, Liu E. Assessment and emergency management of suicidality in personality disorders. Psychiatr Clin North Am. 2008;31(3):527–43.
4. Gabbard GO, Wilkinson SM. Management of countertransference with borderline patients. Washington, DC: American Psychiatric Press; 1994.
5. Richmond JS, Berlin JS, Fishkind AB, et al. Verbal De-escalation of the agitated patient: consensus statement of the American Association for Emergency Psychiatry Project BETA De-escalation Workgroup. West J Emerg Med. 2012;13(1):17–25.
6. Tyrer P, Silk KR. A comparison of UK and US guidelines for drug treatment in borderline personality disorder. Int Rev Psychiatry. 2011;23(4):388–94.
7. Gunderson JG. Borderline personality disorder: a clinical guide: American Psychiatric Publishing, Washington; DC: 2009.

Dr. Hong is a Clinical Assistant Professor of Psychiatry and the Medical Director of the Psychiatric Emergency Services at the University of Michigan. His clinical, educational, and research interests are in the areas of personality disorders, college mental health, and emergency psychiatry. He received his bachelor's degree from the University of California at Berkeley, medical degree from Loma Linda University, and completed his residency at the University of Michigan.

Dr. Bartek is a Clinical Instructor of Psychiatry and the Residency Outpatient Site Director at the University of Michigan. He received his bachelor's degree from Kenyon College, medical degree from the Keck School of Medicine at USC, and completed his residency at the University of Michigan.

Inpatient Psychiatric Management

7

Zeina Saliba

Case Introduction

Dominique is a 32-year-old unemployed domiciled woman, who arrived to the emergency department by ambulance after her boyfriend contacted EMS from home, 5 min after intentional overdose of ten clonazepam tablets, three zolpidem pills, several duloxetine capsules and all that remained in her bottles of clonidine, divalproex and hydrocodone. Poison control was notified and she was admitted to the medicine service, with telemetry monitoring, for observation. Psychiatry was consulted, and you review her records, noting this is her third such presentation to your hospital this year. The patient is on a one-to-one observation status and is eager

Z. Saliba, M.D.
Department of Psychiatry & Behavioral Sciences, George Washington University, Washington, DC, USA

Department of Obstetrics & Gynecology, Virginia Commonwealth University, Richmond, VA, USA
e-mail: zsaliba@gwu.edu

© Springer International Publishing AG, part of Springer Nature 2018
B. Palmer, B. Unruh (eds.), *Borderline Personality Disorder*,
https://doi.org/10.1007/978-3-319-90743-7_7

to speak with you. She describes impulsively taking her prescription medications in an attempt to go to sleep and never wake up, explaining that she "[is] bipolar," and was feeling depressed last week. She tells you that she has insomnia, high blood pressure and was recently diagnosed with fibromyalgia. She feels better since getting to the hospital and requests inpatient admission, noting she is getting "manicky" and does not think she should go home.

Choice Point 1

For each choice point, choose H: "helpful," U: "unhelpful or harmful," or P: "perhaps helpful, with reservations."

In response to Dominique's request for hospitalization, you:

1. Refuse to hospitalize her due to likely harm that may result from hospitalization.
2. Agree to admit her only if you can find a specialized borderline treatment program.
3. Ask her what she expects to gain from hospitalization.
4. Tell her that both of you need to understand more about what led to her overdose to determine what the next steps should be.
5. Agree to hospitalize her after first discussing the possible risks and benefits, length and goal of admission.

Discussion

This patient's overdose was a suicide attempt with moderate lethality and high likelihood of rescue. She has not yet identified any specific preceding stressors, but you appropriately suspect interpersonal stress. The first, and most important, step in assessment is to work with her to develop a narrative of what happened. Did she take the pills one by one? In handfuls? In front of her boyfriend? Was she angry with him? Afraid? What thoughts did she have? Hopes? There is much to understand before moving on to what to do next. If she is unable to engage in that process, then hospitalization may be necessary. (We have a sense that this may be the case here.) Indeed, admission may be necessary regardless, given the severity of the attempt, the frequency of the attempts and the early sense that she is not currently making use of outpatient approaches. While admission may reinforce maladaptive patterns and self-harm behaviors, it may offer a chance to help her understand her reactivity and the process that leads her toward suicide – and develop skills and strategies to more effectively manage her intense emotions. Practically, refusing may escalate risk of further suicidal behavior. At this point, the chronicity of her suicidality and the level of her outpatient services remain unclear, and she may benefit from further evaluation. While a specialized inpatient BPD program may be more helpful than a general unit, it is unlikely you will find one. Option 3 does not explicitly have you committing to a course of action but does have the benefit of asking her to reflect and be an active participant in her care.

Answers

1. U
2. P
3. H
4. H
5. H

Principles and Clinical Pearls

1. It is important to actively involve the patient with BPD in the decision to hospitalize and to base it on an explicit, joint understanding of the potential benefits and likely harm that may result from admission.
2. Hospital stays to deal with crises can be justified, but should be kept short.
3. It is wise to establish a timeframe at point of admission to discourage regressive, idealized, and dependent attachment to the hospital environment.
4. Admission should have specific goals, ideally agreed upon by the patient and clinicians.

Case Continues...

Dominique is transferred to the psychiatric unit (without a sitter) and is interviewed more thoroughly by the inpatient team. She describes herself as having been a normal "moody" teenager. She can enjoy things in her life but has never felt consistently content. She often gets angry, at the drop of a hat – she can be "fine" one minute and upset the next. Other people tell her that she is overreacting, and usually it is due to an external stressor such as a fight with a boyfriend, a negative interaction with her neighbors, or being let down by her family. She has gotten into many fights, even one resulting in jail time. She has been on disability for "manic depression" for four years, before which she had difficulty keeping a job. She denies low self-esteem and feelings of emptiness, explaining that other people just do not understand her; she sometimes feels that people are against her. She has had several suicide attempts but has never cut or burned herself. She is not able to identify any discrete episodes consistent with hypomania or mania, explaining that her doctor told her that her difficulty controlling her moods is because of bipolar disorder, which can make her act impulsively. She smokes marijuana every day, rarely drinks alcohol, and occasionally uses crack cocaine.

Choice Point 2

With regard to diagnosis, you:

1. Suggest reviewing the BPD diagnostic criteria together.
2. Tell her she was misdiagnosed with bipolar and she has BPD.
3. Explore the substance use further, suspecting that there may be active substance use disorder(s).
4. Request contact information for family and outpatient treaters to obtain collateral.
5. Do nothing. She only meets 4 BPD criteria and while you do not think she has bipolar, you do not have an alternative diagnosis that fits.

Discussion

An accurate diagnosis sets up the patient for the most success in treatment and in life. Despite fears about stigma, it is irresponsible not to thoroughly investigate the possibility of BPD. Going over the diagnostic criteria together is a useful method for engaging the patient and building a relationship while clarifying the diagnosis. Choice 2 may be accurate but telling her that without establishing more of a bond may backfire if she thinks you "decided" this too quickly (essentially negating her relationship with her current psychiatrist). Although the substance use may not overtly present as a primary problem, it is important to better understand her patterns of use, as this will greatly influence her prognosis, stability and will guide the appropriate next steps in treatment. Patients with BPD do not always have good insight so getting information from others who know them well can be helpful in establishing a diagnosis. That said, most people with BPD react with appreciation when reviewing criteria that seem to fit their experience better. Choice 5 would be harmful, as strictly adhering to the need for 5 diagnostic criteria will often miss people who will benefit from treatment of BPD.

Answers

1. H
2. P
3. H
4. H
5. U

Principles and Clinical Pearls

1. There is definite clinical value in making and sharing the BPD diagnosis.
2. Inviting the patient to review diagnostic criteria with you, to see if they fit, involves the patient in the process and is alliance building.
3. The presence of any three of the following criteria should make it difficult not to diagnose BPD: excessive anger, interpersonal symptomatology, and self-destructive behaviors.

Case Continues...

You share with her your impression, and after looking over the DSM together, Dominique tells you that it definitely sounds like her. You provide some basic psycho-education and explain that crises and suicidal thoughts are often prompted by interpersonal stress. She tells you that she has not been getting along with her boyfriend but that it is nothing particularly new.

Choice Point 3

You decide to pursue the following next step(s):

1. Push her to reflect further on disagreements with her boyfriend and other possible stressors.
2. With permission, call the boyfriend and ask for his version of events.
3. Comment that the sequelae of overdosing led to her finding relief in a highly structured environment, wondering if structure and care have improved her symptoms.
4. Encourage her to think about aftercare planning.
5. Have the inpatient social worker create a safety contract for Dominique to sign.
6. Instruct Dominique to develop a safety plan for herself, with the social worker's help as needed.

Discussion

The first option involves actively helping the patient to gain more awareness into triggers and interpersonal sensitivity, and make connections between conflict and thoughts of self-harm that will help her learn relevant regulatory strategies to improve future outcomes. Involving families and other support networks (option 2) is an essential component of care. However, at this juncture, helping the patient identify and manage her own emotions and reactions is more important than attempting to establish an objective reality about what happened and who was right or wrong. It is also beneficial to frame their participation accurately and not for the sole purpose of obtaining collateral. The third option is insightful but perhaps better to have her come to this conclusion on her own or with guidance. Although it is possibly too early to start making aftercare plans, it is important to introduce it now. Safety contracts, per se, are unhelpful to the extent that they rely on a commitment that may not be stably present in a crisis and can undermine effective crisis planning. On the other hand, safety planning is an important part of aftercare planning and useful throughout treatment, but again with the patient's active participation in creating and modifying it.

Answers

1. H
2. P
3. P
4. H
5. U
6. H

Principles and Clinical Pearls

1. It is important to encourage self-awareness and involve the patient as an active collaborator, especially in chain analyses.
2. Assume preceding interpersonal stressor(s), such as a rejection (or perception of such), after crisis but clarify precipitants.
3. Changing levels of care can be anxiety provoking, so giving advanced notice and describing next steps promotes a stable transition.
4. Anticipate recurrences – As an exercise, problem solving about alternative coping strategies/methods to manage problems and stress is beneficial and can also produce something tangible for patient to use.

Case Continues...

A short while later, Dominique complains of anxiety and asks for her clonazepam. The nurse tells her that it is not ordered; she gets upset and demands to speak to the doctor.

Choice Point 4

With regard to Dominique's anger about the holding of her benzodiazepine, how would you respond?

1. Explain that she cannot have it yet because she just overdosed on it.
2. Tell the nurse to deal with it because you are busy and do not want to set up unrealistic expectations about your availability.
3. Order a one-time dose of clonazepam.
4. Share your concerns with her about relying on a benzodiazepine to manage her anxiety, and ask her if she has found or can imagine any other helpful anxiolytic strategies.

Discussion

Pharmacologic discussion and management is an important components of inpatient BPD treatment. In this instance, it is reasonable and appropriate to not immediately restart a medication on which she just overdosed, but this is not the complete story. Withholding it entirely during her stay may put her at risk for withdrawal. Giving her what she wants without further exploration of what it means or its role does not help her to build a capacity for tolerating negative emotion, self-soothing, or finding alternative coping skills. This situation provides an opportunity to assess the current effectiveness of her outpatient treatment and review her medication regimen together – likely to be a welcome intervention by the outpatient provider (with whom consultation is absolutely worthwhile). Another important component is to include the nurse in the discussion – to make sure all are on the same page and to minimize future splitting.

Answers

1. P
2. U
3. U
4. H

Principles and Clinical Pearls

1. No medications are FDA approved to treat borderline personality disorder, and caution should be taken in prescribing, with the potential for self-harm taken into account.
2. Requests for medication provide an opportunity for psycho-education and psychopharmacologic education, especially about the limits of effectiveness.
3. Avoid all-or-nothing stances, such as: "this medication is all bad, and it will not help."
4. Asking patients what they think can help foster self-agency.
5. Regular communication between staff members safeguards against splitting.

Case Continues...

She tells you that it is one of the few things that has worked (effectively lowers her anxiety). She does not find divalproex or duloxetine helpful, but she absolutely cannot get to sleep without zolpidem.

Choice Point 5

Anticipating complaints about insomnia tonight, you:

1. Preemptively order PRN trazodone.
2. Let her know that she will still be unable this evening to take the medications she just used in overdose, but you would like to come up with a plan together for addressing her problems of sleeping.
3. Order zolpidem at half the prescribed outpatient dose.
4. Offer the option to ask for diphenhydramine should she have problems falling asleep.
5. Let the nurses and on-call resident deal with it if it becomes an issue.

Discussion

The first choice is relatively safe and could be helpful, but ordering it without discussing her concerns and involving her in the decision-making process is not ideal; the second choice is preferable. Dominique has already expressed that she wants to continue using clonazepam for her anxiety; this can be an opportunity to explain the dangers of using benzodiazepine and nonbenzodiazepine hypnotics together. Although it may not be safe tonight, the third option could be a reasonable compromise (with plan to taper) once it is safe to restart. The fourth option can represent a compromise, whereby you are agreeing to use pharmacologic management for insomnia instead of relying solely on sleep hygiene recommendations, but are also expressing that the type of medication is not negotiable. The last option may seem desirable, especially if you are busy or feeling burnt out, but she has expressed frustration and avoiding it does not model exemplary behavior in regard to confronting charged and potentially uncomfortable situations. It may also make her feel more upset, unheard, blown off and uncared for.

Answers

1. P
2. H
3. P
4. P
5. U

Principles and Clinical Pearls

1. Hypnotic drug therapy has the potential for misuse and is recommended for severe insomnia and short-term use.

2. Prescribing can be done in a way that models effective negotiation between patient and psychiatrist.
3. It is important for patients to be actively involved in finding solutions to their problems.

Case Continues...

She reluctantly agrees to try trazodone, understanding the consequences of overdosing. The next morning she reports having slept just "ok" and having difficulty getting rest because staff kept checking on her and her roommate was snoring. She feels better than when she first came in, attended morning goals group and is looking forward to music therapy this afternoon. She wants to talk about when she can restart her medications and says that you can call her psychiatrist, who will tell you how important it is for her to get them. You plan to speak with her psychiatrist and you tell Dominique that you would also like to contact her therapist, boyfriend and mother, with whom she lives. She refuses permission for these calls and tells you that her therapist is out of town, her boyfriend probably broke up with her after this incident, and talking to her mom will just make things worse.

Choice Point 6

How do you respond?

1. Tell her that you will try to contact her therapist, who may be back.
2. Inquire further about her belief that her mother will escalate the situation.
3. Call her boyfriend and mother without her permission.
4. Explain that this is an expectation of treatment, and nonparticipation could lead to early discharge.
5. Schedule a family meeting, despite her reluctance.

Discussion

This question highlights a common and difficult issue, when the patient either revokes or withholds consent for you to speak with important contacts. Asking her to identify supports is an important step in then bringing them in for psycho-education as well as planning aftercare. She has spontaneously suggested that you speak with her psychiatrist. It is advisable to also be in touch with her therapist, who is also part of her outpatient team and must be included in discharge planning. The therapist may be back from vacation, have set up coverage or have a way for you to leave a message for when they returns. It is important to involve her boyfriend and her mother, as leaving her conflicts with these key supports unaddressed will likely perpetuate recurring sources of interpersonal stress in the outpatient setting.

The question then is how to accomplish this in the face of her refusing to grant permission. There may be legal limitations prohibiting unconsented contact with family and friends at this juncture, whereas upon initial presentation in the emergency department, an argument could be made that contacting them to acquire collateral information is necessary to assist with emergent decision-making. At this point in the case, the goal of contact is extends beyond obtaining information to sharing information about her treatment as well as increasing active involvement. Aside from legal concerns, there is also a risk of alienating the patient and breaking her trust at this early stage. Exploring the patient's resistance can generate opportunities for you to share your perspective and for her to consider it and change her mind, which would be ideal. Staying firm about recommendations, while still allowing patients to make the decisions (and deal with consequences) may be a reasonable compromise. Option 4 is unnecessarily punitive. The last choice could be considered when you have a more established relationship with the patient.

Answers

1. H
2. H
3. U
4. P
5. U

Principles and Clinical Pearls

1. Patients' resistance to involve family members and support persons in aftercare planning should be explored and challenged.
2. Stabilizing relationships with key outpatient supports can lower the risk of repeated hospitalizations.
3. Involve supports in creating safety plans.

Case Continues...

Dominique is scheduled to be discharged back home in two days. You begin to prepare her, asking about what she has learned during hospitalization, reviewing scheduled follow-up appointments and identifying what remains to be planned. You ask her to look over her outpatient safety plan and meet with the social worker this afternoon. The next morning the nurses report that she was found in her room last night scratching herself with a plastic dinner fork. They added a 1:1 sitter.

Choice Point 7

How do you respond to this behavior?

1. Delay the discharge date by another week.
2. Help her realize she is seeking caregiving and attention.
3. Consider PHP or IOP instead of returning to standard outpatient care.
4. Continue with planned discharge date.
5. Ask about her intentions, why she did this.

Discussion

Patients often have regressive or even angry reactions when stepping down from higher levels of care, even when involved in discharge planning. It is important to follow through agreed-upon discharge timelines, unless there is evidence that she cannot make use of outpatient supports or you assess a high level of dangerousness to be present (not clearly present in this case). Delaying her discharge date does not hold Dominique accountable nor help her gain skills to cope with discomfort. She may not understand why she did this, as patients are often unaware of underlying motivations and bringing them to light can be helpful. If not already planned, option 3 is ideal because it organizes a stepwise progression from a setting of high security and structure to one that fosters more independence.

Answers

1. U
2. P
3. H
4. H
5. P

Principles and Clinical Pearls

1. As discharge date approaches, expect patients to experience anxiety; You should anticipate regression.
2. Minimize such reactions by decreasing from a maximal to minimal level of structure across therapeutic and other functions.
3. Decreasing levels of support in a stepwise fashion is ideal.

Summary of Clinical Approach

Key principles of inpatient management are reviewed and are consistent with many basic lessons from other levels of care. First, it is important to hospitalize reluctantly, differentiating nonlethal from true suicidal intent and searching for least restrictive safe option. Decision to hospitalize should ideally involve the patient (clearly presenting risk of destabilization) and outpatient team. When hospitalization is recommended, shorter stays are almost always preferable to longer term, which may easily become regressive. It can be helpful to point out the unconscious desire to be cared for, in the safety provided by the structured holding environment. Taking responsibility for patients' needs in times of crisis may inadvertently undermine their capacity to care for themselves. The goals may include keeping the patient safe, exploring antecedent incidents, providing education, evaluating current treatment (approach as well as medication regimen), planning transition to aftercare and including the patient and family in the various steps. Challenges often present themselves around team splitting, family contact and increasing anxiety at time of planned discharge. Helping the patient modulate emotions through this process will be beneficial in modeling behaviors that she/he can use outside of the hospital.

> **Clinician Experience: Leading Inpatient Teams**
> Inpatient clinicians face specific challenges when leading teams of mental health professionals likely to have divergent opinions about BPD patients. Staff are prone to become overly supportive or overly punitive, and patients may quickly become swept up in a question of which staff did or said what. Team leaders are most effective when they can notice and validate the experience of staff – all of whom are conveying a grain of wisdom with their observation that the patient needs more support or stricter limits. Re-orienting staff and the patient to specific goals for the day and goals for the stay can mitigate the splitting and regression that sometimes accompanies hospitalization.

Suggested Readings

1. Gunderson JG. Borderline personality disorder a clinical guide. Washington, DC: American Psychiatric Publishing; 2008.
2. Gunderson JG. Handbook of good psychiatric management for borderline personality disorder. 2014. Washington, DC: American Psychiatric Publishing; 2008.
3. Miller LJ. Inpatient management of borderline personality disorder: a review and update. J Personal Disord. 1989;3(2):122–34.
4. The NICE guideline on treatment & management: borderline personality disorder. National Collaborating Centre for Mental Health: The British Psychological Society and The Royal College of Psychiatrists, 2009. https://www.nice.org.uk/guidance/cg78. Accessed 6/23/18.
5. Practice guidelines for the treatment of patients with borderline personality disorder. American Psychiatric Association. 2001, 2010.

Dr. Saliba is a board-certified psychiatrist, family medicine physician, and addictionologist. She is an Assistant Professor at the George Washington University and the Inpatient Medical Director for Psychiatric & Behavioral Services, overseeing the mental health unit and consultation services. She attended the University of Virginia, the Medical College of Virginia and completed a joint residency at the University of Pittsburgh, where she participated in the Academic Administrator Clinician Educator and Global Health tracks and served as Chief Resident. She is passionate about and dedicated to women's and maternal-child health, decreasing stigma in mental illness and providing care for marginalized populations. Her current efforts are devoted to health equity in the urban setting, refugee health domestically and abroad, partnering with patients and interdisciplinary teaching.

Consultation/Liaison Management in the General Hospital

8

Stephanie H. Cho

Choice Point Index
1. Making the BPD diagnosis in the medical setting
2. Rolling with resistance to the diagnosis and addressing conflict
3. Keeping the big picture in view regarding treatment
4. Responding to distress and suicidal comments
5. Responding to requests for psychiatric hospitalization

Case Introduction

The inpatient medical service requests a psychiatric consultation on a "non-compliant" patient. Sally is a 56-year-old woman with longstanding blood pressure and cholesterol problems who was admitted to the hospital for chest pain. The medical team informs you that Sally's chest pain was not a heart attack as initially thought, but rather exertional angina due to a combination of stress and not taking her medications. When told that she is at high risk for heart attack due to her poor adherence to her medications, Sally became upset and started yelling, saying "I knew you would find a way to blame me! Just like everyone else!" The medical team also mentioned that Sally has been a "challenging" patient and was often irritable with staff. Aware of your concern that the medical team may have requested your consultation due to dislike of the patient, you go interview Sally.

During consultation, you learn that Sally has been feeling angry and depressed since her husband filed for divorce. She stops taking her medications when she feels that "there is no point when everyone I love hates me." She was brought to the hospital after developing chest pain during a fight with her daughter who "took her

_____

S. H. Cho, M.D., M.S.
Department of Psychiatry and Behavioral Sciences, Keck School of Medicine of the
University of Southern California, Los Angeles, CA, USA

© Springer International Publishing AG, part of Springer Nature 2018   89
B. Palmer, B. Unruh (eds.), *Borderline Personality Disorder*,
https://doi.org/10.1007/978-3-319-90743-7_8

father's side." During the remainder of the consultation, Sally tells you that she has always been "moody," with episodes of depression and a history of multiple over-doses (none of which required medical treatment). She did not finish college due to problems with alcohol, but became sober during pregnancy. Sally and her husband have had many separations during their marriage, during which she would relapse on alcohol. She superficially cut for many years when distressed but has stopped in recent years. Sally complained that, except for the cardiologist, "no one here seems to know what they're doing."

Choice Point 1

For each choice point, choose H: "helpful," U: "unhelpful or harmful," or P: "per-haps helpful, with reservations."

You feel confident in the diagnosis of borderline personality disorder. Would you:

1. Disclose the diagnosis to Sally and provide psychoeducation on the etiology, course, and prognosis.
2. Avoid discussing the diagnosis with Sally to prevent further destabilization dur-ing her hospitalization.
3. Disclose the diagnosis to Sally's medical team and provide psychoeducation to better prepare them to interact with Sally.
4. Carefully avoid mentioning BPD to Sally and the medical team, as disclosure would only worsen the relationship between Sally and her doctors by increasing stigmatization and shame.

Discussion

People with BPD have higher rates of chronic illness, pain, and utilization of health-care resources[1], accounting for 10–15% of emergency room visits[2] and 6% of primary care visits[3]. Borderline personality also accounts for a significant portion, if not the majority, of personality disorders seen by consulting psychiatric ser-vices[4]. Consultation psychiatrists are frequently the first to diagnose BPD and should inform and educate the patient about the disorder, as in Choice 1. The inter-personal difficulties that are central to BPD negatively impact relationships with healthcare professionals, contributing to poor quality of care and health[5]. Making patients aware that their interpersonal difficulties stem from a treatable condition offers them hope and the opportunity to pursue treatment to mitigate these effects and more successfully manage their medical conditions[1].

In the general hospital setting, educating other healthcare providers about BPD can be of substantial benefit. While some people with medical illnesses can regress, a history of unstable relationships, abandonment fears, and impulsive self-harm and suicidal behaviors should raise reasonable certainty that the BPD diagnosis is accurate and should be made. Unrecognized BPD can incite negative reactions in clinicians that hinder patient care (see "Clinician Experience" sidebar). Awareness of the diagnosis, as well as improved understanding of the psychological underpinnings of BPD, enables clinicians to set realistic expectations for treatment, recognize motivations (often unconscious) driving provocations, and better manage their own emotions (Choice 3).

Consulting psychiatrists may hesitate to disclose a diagnosis of BPD for a variety of reasons. Some may be concerned that the diagnosis would instill destabilizing shame or rejection, as in Choice 2, or intensify stigmatization from treating providers, as in Choice 4. However, concealing the diagnosis would further perpetuate stigma. It is also possible that these concerns are more a reflection of the consultant's own anxieties regarding BPD.

Answers

1. H
2. U
3. H
4. U

Principles and Clinical Pearls

1. Diagnostic disclosure and psychoeducation can improve care and communication by establishing realistic expectations and enabling both patients and clinicians to interact more effectively.
2. Disclosing the diagnosis during non-psychiatric hospitalization is an opportunity to engage intreatment patients who might otherwise remain undiagnosed.
3. Effective BPD treatment increases the likelihood of successfully managing other medical conditions.

Case Continues...

You ask Sally for permission to discuss your thoughts. She consents and you proceed to review the diagnostic criteria of BPD with her. Sally agrees that the criteria aptly describe her life. However, when you name borderline personality disorder, she vehemently disagrees with your diagnosis. Suddenly upset, she yells "I thought you were different from the other doctors, that you actually cared. Instead you just call me borderline!" She further complains that you make this "accusation" when you "don't even know me!"

Choice Point 2

How would you respond to Sally's reaction to your assessment?

1. Reiterate the diagnosis, supporting your assessment by connecting diagnostic criteria to information she shared with you.
2. "This isn't an accusation. Why would you think that?"
3. "I can tell that you are upset. Can you help me understand what I did to upset you?"
4. "You have some strong feelings about "borderline." What does "borderline" mean to you?"
5. Apologize and internally make a note that Sally does not have enough insight to accept her diagnosis.

Discussion

Sally's outrage is an example of the interpersonal hypersensitivity that is characteristic of BPD. When threatened by perceived hostility or criticism, anxiety and fear of rejection drives borderline patients to seek help and reassurance in maladaptive ways, including devaluation, self-injury, and anger. In this case, Sally likely interpreted the BPD diagnosis as blaming her for the problems she experiences. Patients in non-psychiatric settings may interpret a BPD diagnosis as minimization or rejection of their "real" physical complaints. In these episodes of distress, the consultant should first acknowledge the distress to let the patient know they have been "heard." To reassure the patient that the consultant is present and interested, one should first express concern and curiosity. After reducing the patient's reactivity, the consultant can explore the reason for distress, encouraging reflection and introspection. Here the consultant has the opportunity to build trust and engage the patient.

Choices 3 and 4 both acknowledge the patient's distress, but explore it from different perspectives. Choice 2 indirectly acknowledges Sally's distress in a defensive rather than supportive manner that could be interpreted as further rejection. Choice 1 would likely further anger and alienate Sally. Rather than exploring Sally's resistance to the diagnosis, Choice 5 prematurely judges Sally's ability to cope and accept her diagnosis.

Answers

1. U
2. P
3. H
4. H
5. U

Principles and Clinical Pearls

1. Acknowledging emotional distress can reduce reactivity by allowing the borderline patient to feel "heard."
2. Expressing concerned curiosity reassures patients that the consultant is present, interested, and engaged.
3. Exploring emotional responses engages the patient in reflection and introspection while building trust.

Case Continues...

Calmer, but still suspicious, Sally tells you that she has "known some borderlines, they're selfish and dramatic" and that she is nothing like them. She feels the borderline diagnosis places blame on her for the family conflict and its negative impact on her health. You agree that these are hurtful thoughts and tell her that your intention was not to blame, but rather to highlight how these struggles could be symptoms of the disorder. Sally accepts that you did not mean to offend but still expresses disagreement with the diagnosis.

Choice Point 3

How would you respond to Sally's continued rejection of the borderline diagnosis?

1. Drop the issue completely, with no intention to revisit the discussion as it will only cause further negative reaction and sabotage any possible progress.
2. Gently maintain your diagnostic impression, but acknowledge that you do not know her well and could be wrong. Move the discussion to treatment strategies that are informed by the diagnosis without further debating it.
3. Ask, "How do you feel I could be most helpful?"

Discussion

Working effectively with borderline patients requires practicality and flexibility. As with other diagnoses, insistence on "being right" can cause significant harm and risks completely alienating the patient. With their underlying hypersensitivity, borderline patients are particularly prone to withdraw and reject in such situations. The patient is better served if the consultant can adjust to the patient's needs, "agree to disagree," and instead focus on identifying treatment goals that the patient can accept. Choice 2 maintains the consultant's assessment while simultaneously reassuring the patient that she is being heard and her opinion is considered. This response has the additional benefit of modeling tolerance of uncertainty and admission of fallibility, both of which are difficult for borderline patients.

Choice 1 is over-reactive and likely reflects the consultant's own anxiety around giving the diagnosis and low expectations for improvement. The discussion should be revisited in the future as there are still benefits for accepting the diagnosis. Choice 3 alone does not address the patient's objection and could be interpreted as rejection or withdrawal. It would be better combined with Choice 2.

Answers

1. U
2. H
3. P

Principles and Clinical Pearls

1. Flexibility and practicality are the key to effectively work with BPD.
2. Used judiciously, "agreeing to disagree" can help maintain therapeutic alliance, while also modeling important skills such as compromise and tolerance.
3. Admitting fallibility and uncertainty can strengthen the consultant's authenticity and counter "black and white" thinking.

Case Continues...

Sally is surprised by your willingness to admit uncertainty about her diagnosis, but unsure how you can help her. You note that the consultation was requested due to concern about Sally's adherence to medication and tell Sally that you are concerned stress is severely limiting her ability to care for her health. She agrees but does not know how to fix it, claiming "that's just what happens when I get stressed out." You suggest that developing additional ways to manage stress could improve her ability to manage her illness, and you draw her attention to the relationships in her life that fuel her stress, wondering if she stops medications (and thinks of dying) when she fears being left alone. You work with Sally to identify some coping skills that were helpful in the past and recommend she begin psychotherapy after discharge. With her consent, you make arrangements for her to follow up with an outpatient clinician.

The next morning you receive a call from Sally's nurse who tells you that Sally has become agitated, verbally abusive and out of control. The medical team had informed Sally that she would be discharged later in the day with instructions to restart her home medications and follow up with her regular doctor. When you arrive at Sally's room, she is furious, saying she is not well enough to be discharged, and "They're just trying to get rid of me because they don't like me!" She then bursts out crying, saying "No one cares about me, not even doctors! I might as well be dead!"

Choice Point 4

How do you respond to Sally's outburst?

1. Ask the medical team to delay discharge.
2. Admit Sally to a psychiatric unit to ensure safety — involuntarily if necessary.
3. Recommend the medical team discharge Sally to avoid rewarding her manipulative gestures, and inform Sally that she will be discharged.
4. Express concern about her obvious distress and ask to discuss it.
5. Perform an extensive and detailed suicide risk evaluation.

Discussion

Borderline patients do have an increased risk of suicide, and the risk is further elevated in those who engage in self-harm. Therefore, self-harm should prompt an assessment of the patient's risk of actual dangerousness. The consultant's reaction at this stage is critical. The consultant should actively express concern, but avoid becoming reactive. Better yet, the consultant should help the patient grow more active in considering how to mitigate her risk on discharge with increased structure, skill use, and appropriate connection with outpatient treatment. Consultants unfamiliar with the underlying fears and insecurities associated with BPD may respond with anger or withdrawal that will worsen the patient's distress and increase physical danger. Conversely, the consultant may over-react and inadvertently reinforce the use of these behaviors. Consultants with a better understanding of BPD hypersensitivity could view Sally's emotional response in context of the threat of abandonment posed by discharge, and thus be better prepared to provide support to calm and de-escalate. As discussed earlier, acknowledging the patient's feelings in a non-reactive manner while expressing concern and curiosity would be the most effective response (Choice 4).

Choices 1 and 2 are over-reactions that may validate Sally's perceived rejection, reinforce the use of suicidal threats, and ultimately worsen her condition. In this case, losing the support and containment afforded by hospitalization has activated Sally's fears of abandonment. For this reason, prolonged or frequent hospitalizations can become harmful and should be used only if necessary to maintain safety. In Choice 5, conducting an extensive suicide risk assessment without first gauging the actual level of risk is also an over-reaction and may paradoxically be harmful by inserting the verbalizing suicidal urges would get her needs met. A reasonable approach could include taking seriously her concerns (agreeing that the discharge will leave her lonely) and encouraging her to redouble efforts to incorporate skills and structure while assessing (and documenting) her levels of internal agitation, future orientation, hopelessness, and distress. Her discharge plan should include increased daytime structure to mitigate the increased risk of suicide due to transitioning to a lower level of care. Choice 3 fails to assess actual dangerousness in addition to being punitive and retaliatory, which could drive Sally further toward self-harm.

Answers

1. U
2. U
3. U
4. H
5. P

Principles and Pearls

1. Anticipating an increase in symptoms with a transition to a lower level of care can help prepare both the patient and treatment team for the need for increased structure and support during the post-hospital period.
2. Considering a borderline patient's emotional reaction to threat can better enable the consultant to provide support in a non-reactive, concerned, and curious manner.
3. Withdrawal or punitive responses worsen patients' distress and increase the risk of harm, while over-reaction can validate distorted perceptions of threat and reinforce maladaptive behaviors.

Case Continues...

After further discussion with Sally, you feel confident that her risk of actually harming herself is low. The medical team enters the room and insists that Sally be admitted to the psychiatric hospital for suicidal thoughts since she no longer requires hospitalization for her chest pain. Before you can answer, Sally quickly agrees, insisting that psychiatric hospitalization is the "best thing" for her.

Choice Point 5

How would you respond to Sally's request for psychiatric hospitalization?

1. Agree to hospitalization despite your belief that it will reinforce manipulative and avoidant behaviors.
2. Refuse to hospitalize Sally based on your low concern for self-harm.
3. Ask Sally why she feels psychiatric hospitalization is the "best thing" for her.
4. Tell her that you may have to reluctantly support hospitalization for fear she will grow more suicidal if you do not, but share your concern that psychiatric hospitalization will not be helpful and may actually make it harder for her to eventually transition home; instead, suggest she work on a plan for increased structure and crisis management ("Wouldn't that be a better plan?").

5. Discuss alternative treatment options such as intensive outpatient or partial hospitalization programs.

Discussion

In the case that a patient desires hospitalization for suicidality but the consultant does not consider it appropriate, rigid refusal may intensify the risk of a suicidal event while capitulation can reinforce the maladaptive behavior. Here again, flexibility and pragmatism should be exercised as the consultant continues to maintain concern and curiosity while keeping the patient's safety the priority. Choice 4 acknowledges the patient's distress and maintains the consultant's recommendation while compromising if necessary to ensure the patient's safety. Choice 3 engages the patient to explore their desire for hospitalization. Together, Choices 3 and 4 keep the patient in an active role, managing her own safety and decisions with consultation and input from her treaters.

Choice 5 could be helpful in educating the patient on other options, but could also be interpreted as minimizing or ignoring the patient's distress. Choice 1 exemplifies the consultant's preference to avoid angering the patient and other clinicians. Non-psychiatric clinicians may request or even insist on inpatient psychiatric hospitalization to alleviate their own anxieties as well as to free themselves of the challenges of a borderline patient. However, the psychiatric consultant should mitigate the effects of these recommendations and champion what is best for the patient. Unyielding refusal without discussion, as in Choice 2, can lead to dangerous escalation of the patient's distress.

Answers

1. U
2. U
3. H
4. H
5. P

Principles and Pearls

1. Response to the patient in crisis remains rooted in acknowledging emotional distress, expressing concern, and exploring the emotional response.
2. Flexibility and pragmatism are the key to effectively working with borderline patients.
3. Recommendation against hospitalization can be communicated as an appeal to use skills, structure, and agency to manage a difficult period—appealing to the patient's courage and helping avoid passivity.

Summary of Clinical Approach

This case demonstrates basic principles of working with BPD as employed by the psychiatric consultant in the general hospital setting. Diagnostic disclosure establishes appropriate expectations for treatment and may improve patient and clinician interaction. Effective consultants are flexible and practical, reassuring to the patient while at the same time containing reactivity and encouraging introspection. Finally, this case highlights the vital role psychiatric consultants play in improving quality of care for borderline patients through crisis intervention and liaison efforts.

Clinician Experience: Impulse to Punish or Abandon

Patients with BPD incite strong, often negative, emotions in clinicians, including incompetence (after devaluation), powerlessness (after attack), or feeling exploited (after manipulation). These emotions can lead clinicians to react in two ways: withdrawal and retaliation. Clinicians who withdraw from the patient may avoid, neglect, or even abandon the patient. Others may retaliate, employ punitive measures, and blame or shame patients through inappropriate confrontations. These emotions and subsequent reactions are often jarring, contrary as they are to the caretaker identity of most clinicians. Abandonment or retaliation by the clinician also aggravates the underlying insecurities and fears of the borderline patient.

Fortunately, these harms can be prevented. While against the clinician's nature, the clinician must first recognize without shame or self-blame that the patient evokes these feelings. Once aware, the clinician can reflect and appreciate how underlying fears of abandonment and rejection drive the behaviors that evoke such negative feelings. This realization can be a normalizing experience, both destigmatizing the clinician's feelings and making the patient's difficult behaviors more comprehensible. This improved understanding enables the clinician to take steps to adjust their own reactions and behaviors, in a way modeling the very self-regulatory processes one would ask of the borderline patient.

In non-psychiatric settings, psychiatric consultations are usually requested after patients have been labeled "difficult" and clinicians are already acting on their negative emotions. It falls to the psychiatric consultant to educate other providers on BPD, help them identify behavioral conflicts that are likely to arise, help them adjust their actions to more effectively care for these patients, and provide a space to air and process their negative emotions.

References and Recommended Reading

1. Frankenburg FR, Zanarini MC. The association between borderline personality disorder and chronic medical illnesses, poor health-related lifestyle choices, and costly forms of health care utilization. J Clin Psychiatry. 2004;65(12):1660–5. http://www.ncbi.nlm.nih.gov/pubmed/15641871.
2. Tomko RL, Trull TJ, Wood PK, Sher KJ. Characteristics of borderline personality disorder in a community sample: comorbidity, treatment utilization, and general functioning. J Personal Disord. 2014;28(5):734–50. https://doi.org/10.1521/pedi_2012_26_093.
3. Gross R, Olfson M, Gameroff M. Borderline personality disorder in primary care. Arch Intern Med. 2002;162(1):53–60. https://doi.org/10.1001/archinte.162.1.53.
4. Laugharne R, Flynn A. Personality disorders in consultation-liaison psychiatry. Curr Opin Psychiatry. 2013;26(1):84–9. https://doi.org/10.1097/YCO.0b013e328359977f.
5. Tyrer P, Reed GM, Crawford MJ. Classification, assessment, prevalence, and effect of personality disorder. Lancet (London, England). 2015;385(9969):717–26. https://doi.org/10.1016/S0140-6736(14)61995-4.
6. Groves JE. Taking care of the hateful patient. N Engl J Med. 1978;298(16):883–7. https://doi.org/10.1056/NEJM197804202981605.
7. Ricke AK, Lee M-J, Chambers JE. The difficult patient. Obstet Gynecol Surv. 2012;67(8):495–502. https://doi.org/10.1097/OGX.0b013e318267f1db.
8. Dubovsky AN, Kiefer MM. Borderline personality disorder in the primary care setting. Med Clin North Am. 2014;98(5):1049–64. https://doi.org/10.1016/j.mcna.2014.06.005.
9. Riddle M, Meeks T, Alvarez C, Dubovsky A. When personality is the problem: managing patients with difficult personalities on the acute care unit. J Hosp Med. 2016;11(12):873–8. https://doi.org/10.1002/jhm.2643.

Dr. Cho is completing her fellowship in Consultation-Liaison Psychiatry at LAC+USC Medical Center in Los Angeles. Her clinical interests focus on improving care for vulnerable and stigmatized populations including borderline personality, somatic symptom disorders, and hospitalized patients with psychiatric disorders. She has a passion for teaching and has been involved in psychiatric education for both psychiatric and non-psychiatric providers at all levels of practice. She has incorporated GPM into the didactic curriculum of residents at LAC+USC Medical Center and plans to integrate GPM principles into the C-L psychiatry services as well. Upon completion of her fellowship, she will be joining the Consultation-Liaison Psychiatry faculty at the University of Southern California Keck School of Medicine.

Substance Use Comorbidities

9

Carl Fleisher

Choice Point Index
1. Addressing drug use early in a treatment.
2. Considering medication for anxiety in a patient with BPD and a substance use disorder.
3. Addressing drug use in an established treatment.
4. Managing impulsivity in early sobriety.
5. Validating experience while simultaneously raising concerns.

Case Introduction

Melissa is a 19-year-old woman who established care with you two months ago after a fall off of a fire escape while under the influence of drugs and alcohol. The fall left her with fractures in her leg and wrist requiring surgical repair. Her parents are divorced. They still argue, though both are trying to make sure that their daughter stays safe. You delivered the diagnosis of borderline personality disorder (BPD) and undertook treatment, anticipating some challenges. Melissa saw the diagnosis of borderline personality disorder as accurate yet was reluctant to pursue treatment because she is only bothered by "anxiety." She manages this using marijuana daily. You provided psycho-education to both parents and referred them to a Family Connections group. Dad found this very helpful, but mom lost touch. Mom's behavior seemed to fit with Melissa's sense of her mother as having always been overwhelmed, unable to tolerate her own or others' emotions to any degree. Melissa experienced her father in childhood as intrusive and often becoming enraged; he has not acted like that around you, however.

C. Fleisher, M.D.
UCLA, Department of Psychiatry and Biobehavioral Sciences, Los Angeles, CA, USA
e-mail: cfleisher@mednet.ucla.edu

© Springer International Publishing AG, part of Springer Nature 2018
B. Palmer, B. Unruh (eds.), *Borderline Personality Disorder*,
https://doi.org/10.1007/978-3-319-90743-7_9

As you move forward in treatment, your frequent efforts to see things from her point of view help her feel understood, and she begins to trust you. She resumes classes at a community college, and her grades rise from Fs to Cs. She is honest about ongoing marijuana use, sometimes smoking before classes begin, yet resists your suggestion that she cut back. She has never been high or intoxicated during therapy, but her grades fall short of her previous scholastic performance.

Choice Point 1

For each choice point, choose H: "helpful," U: "unhelpful or harmful," or P: "perhaps helpful, with reservations".
    With regard to Melissa's frequent marijuana use, you should:

1. Insist that you cannot treat her unless she stops using.
2. Leave it alone, she needs more therapy first.
3. Refer her to a 12-step program.
4. Wonder about and explore whether emotional or interpersonal changes precipitate her use.
5. Ask her parents to start drug-testing her at home to enforce sobriety.

Discussion

The treatment is just getting started. Melissa is beginning to trust your helpful intentions, but marijuana use threatens to derail her initial improvement on several counts. Her past use played a role in her serious physical injury, for one thing. In addition, her current use enables avoidance of emotions that are difficult to manage, and may also reduce her motivation to address interpersonal stressors that engender those emotions. Further avoidance of confronting core emotional and interpersonal problems is likely to hamper interpersonal and academic success, which would otherwise bolster her self-esteem and career opportunities.

    Insisting that she stop using marijuana immediately is an authoritarian stance that is likely to drive her out of treatment. She may not be ready to stop – she has not shown the skills to achieve sobriety or to sustain it. Moreover, it may be more accurate to frame her use as a symptom of her BPD, and from that standpoint, cessation of drug use would not be a precondition of treatment, any more than emotional control would be.

    To say that Melissa needs more therapy before targeting marijuana use raises questions about what else should be targeted, and for how long. A recommendation for psychotherapy for BPD should propose specific goals and methods. You may delay addressing marijuana use if you determine that you need to establish trust more firmly. Otherwise, marijuana use is the most pressing therapeutic target in the case as presented. If you rely on therapy to address her use indirectly (or ignore the use), Melissa may not learn what drives her use, nor have an opportunity to learn coping skills that are more adaptive. Sometimes, we as clinicians assume that patients are too fragile to handle certain interventions, but if she is too fragile for an explicit goal to reduce drug use, then outpatient therapy may not be an appropriate level of care to begin with. You should state clearly that achieving sobriety will be one of your aims for her treatment.

Referral to a 12-step program is a reasonable effort at developing her support network, although there is a dearth of research on interventions for comorbid substance use [1, 2]. It is also preferable to encourage Melissa to be curious about what circumstances precipitate use. At first, you might hear only about external, interpersonal circumstances – finding something that belonged to an ex-boyfriend, perhaps. You will want to link these external events as often as possible to internal reactions, for example, a return of feeling unwanted, or alone. Clarifying these internal states is key to understand how she ends up deciding that marijuana is the best, or only, way to manage, rather than distract herself or seek out friends.

Asking Melissa's parents to perform at-home drug testing may be tempting because it addresses the issue head on, but on reflection, poses several problems. Involving Melissa's parents in this way impedes her agency, that is, her sense of playing an active role in her own life. Borderline personality disorder is characterized by impaired agency, so interventions that further reduce it may be counterproductive over the long-term. Another problem is Melissa's view of her parents as intrusive to begin with. Assigning a policing role to her parents is likely to reinforce that view, rather than give them opportunities to show caring motives and behavior. In addition, in light of Melissa's high likelihood of use with even the best of intentions, drug testing by anyone sets her up for predictable, repeated experiences of failure and shame.

Answers

1. U
2. P
3. P
4. H
5. U

Principles and Clinical Pearls

1. In patients with BPD, it is often useful to frame drug use (or other risky behavior) as an attempt to manage intense emotions, before considering it as an issue separate from BPD.
2. Direct, collaborative discussion of drug use is preferable to punitive or controlling approaches.
3. Drug use, when significant, can be a comorbid disorder that requires its own treatment. Referral to a 12-step program can be an effective first step in addressing problematic use.

Case Continues...

At an early session, you raise your concern about Melissa's use of marijuana. You inquire whether marijuana functions as an escape from intolerable emotions. You also point out how such behavior might slow her treatment progress. Melissa acknowledges that marijuana enables her to participate in social gatherings that she might otherwise avoid and sometimes helps her fall asleep. She says that she has tried medicines for her anxiety, but nothing except marijuana seems to help. She would like to stop using it, though. She wonders whether you might prescribe her something for the anxiety so she will not need marijuana anymore.

Choice Point 2

How would you respond to Melissa's request for medication targeting anxiety?

1. Prescribe a selective serotonin reuptake inhibitor (SSRI), as these agents are first-line pharmacotherapy for social anxiety.
2. Keep medication in mind, but begin by probing for detail about what feelings she would have in social gatherings if she did not use marijuana.
3. Address anxiety in therapy, but prescribe a sedating medication for insomnia.
4. Stop therapy for BPD and refer her to cognitive-behavioral therapy (CBT), the first-line treatment for anxiety.
5. Acknowledge the difficulty in her situation, wanting to sleep restfully and maintain social ties while feeling unable to do so without mind-altering substances.

Discussion

Melissa struggles with a feeling she describes as "anxiety," with interpersonal avoidance significant enough to drive her to use marijuana. Her description thus far is nonspecific, as it may involve feeling flustered in the presence of so many minds that she cannot understand, feeling inadequate, feeling angry that she is not receiving all the attention she wants, or a host of other possibilities. It is important to ask about the specific thoughts and feelings she has, rather than assume that social anxiety (i.e., thoughts that she will be judged or criticized) is present. Exploring Melissa's experience in depth will also serve to illuminate the links between her internal states and other people's behavior.

Even if Melissa does have comorbid social anxiety disorder, BPD should be the primary focus of treatment [3]. Thus, treating social anxiety with CBT is not likely to be effective at this stage. An SSRI might reduce anxiety, but is not likely to be as effective as it would be in the absence of BPD. Prescribing medication for insomnia is reasonable, especially if sleep hygiene strategies have been taught, tried, and found insufficient. If effective, a hypnotic might at least lead her to use marijuana less often.

Regardless of what other choice you make, it is meaningful to acknowledge at least that Melissa is using marijuana to try to achieve valid aims. This will help her feel understood. In general, even though people with borderline personality disorder may act against their long-term self-interest, their behavior often makes sense within the context of their efforts to solve meaningful problems. Appreciating that point not only strengthens rapport but also may reduce the patient's own criticism about his or her own behavior. Overall, the result is to reframe the therapy in the direction of manageable problem solving.

Answers

1. U
2. H
3. P
4. U
5. H

Principles and Clinical Pearls

1. It is critical to have a detailed understanding of how people with BPD arrive at the views they hold. Assumptions about feelings or unscrutinized acceptance of vague emotional descriptions may cloud an opportunity for therapeutic progress, and may even take treatment in an unhelpful direction.
2. It is a common misconception that treatment for comorbid disorders like social anxiety or recurrent depression should take precedence over treatment for BPD. Rather, BPD should be viewed as the primary target of treatment [3].
3. Seeking a genuine appreciation for why a person engages in unhealthy behavior can be more productive than, and often must precede, trying to introduce alternative behaviors.

Case Continues...

You continue working with Melissa on understanding and tolerating the emotions that make social situations difficult to get through without marijuana. Her grades rise to straight Cs. She is able to cut back on marijuana use at bedtime. Despite a period of relative stability in her interpersonal life, however, Melissa continues to use marijuana frequently. She reveals that she has been needing to use more to get the same high, her use sometimes gets out of control, and she has cravings. She skipped two classes last week because she was high. She still socializes primarily with friends who are using marijuana or other drugs. Noticing that Melissa's symptoms meet sufficient criteria to warrant a diagnosis of substance use disorder, you refer her to a local 12-step group. However, Melissa declines. She says that she can stop whenever she needs to. Moreover, now that you have helped reduce her anxiety, she is satisfied with her current grades and social functioning.

Choice Point 3

How would you respond to Melissa's refusal to join a 12-step group?

1. Revisit her goals for treatment.
2. Consider increasing the frequency of visits.
3. Consider reducing treatment until she agrees to address this issue.
4. Agree to put aside talking about substance use for a specific period of time.
5. Try to engage her in understanding your perspective on the risks of use.

Discussion

Now that you have a working relationship with Melissa, you can address her substance use. To do otherwise risks sending the message that you do not think she is capable of such progress, or that she cannot expect any better for herself.

A return to treatment goals (and values) will provide context for whatever discussion may follow. If, for example, she has career goals that would require abstinence from marijuana, you can seek opportunities to link her current choices with those more distant career goals. Increasing the frequency of visits, or adding new treatment modalities, may then help her progress. If, on the other hand, neither Melissa's goals nor her values pertain to marijuana use, her motivation to change that behavior will be low. In that case, you may seek to nurture new goals in alignment with treatment for substance misuse. An impasse could arise if you feel strongly that marijuana use is a barrier to Melissa's own treatment goals, yet she does not see it that way. At that point, you have established a relationship strong enough that you can challenge her, for example by making further treatment contingent on pursuing substance use interventions. This strategy, if simply announced as an edict, risks a weakening of the patient–provider relationship. However, if a contingency is introduced and explained as a starting point for each of you to listen to the point of view of the other, a powerful message is sent: you care about her well-being, you see her as capable of change, and you believe she should seriously consider your recommendation.

Throughout any discussion of goals, it is important to assess Melissa's understanding of both the benefits and risks of her marijuana use. If she is not aware of certain risks, then educate her. If she discounts risk while in the throes of black-and-white thinking, be wary of getting caught in an argument. Search for elements of her view to validate first, and only then try to introduce your own perspective. Introducing alternate perspectives before validating is likely to be experienced by patients with BPD as dismissal or attack. Such a reaction elicits defensiveness and reduces openness to feedback from others.

Answers

1. H
2. P
3. P
4. U
5. H

Principles and Clinical Pearls

1. Treatment recommendations should be guided by the patient's goals, to maximize motivation for change
2. Titrating the intensity and frequency of treatment is an effective intervention when used thoughtfully and with patient input.
3. Ignoring or setting aside an important problem after rapport is established risks stagnation of treatment, or worse, colluding with a reduction of agency and self-esteem.

Case Continues...

You continue discussing Melissa's marijuana use over the next several sessions. At first, she holds fast to her decision to decline substance use treatment. You teach her about the cognitive effects of frequent use, information of which she was not fully aware. With persistent, empathic challenge, she acknowledges that her goal to become a surgeon ultimately depends on sharply reducing her use. She begins to attend Marijuana Anonymous meetings. She finds a sponsor who is 15 years sober. Slowly, some of her grades rise to Bs.

A few weeks later, Melissa comes to a session furious. She explains that her parents have canceled her credit cards. She criticizes them and devalues them at length, revealing only toward the end of the session that the abrupt action came after she spent $7000 on shoes in the past month. "It doesn't matter if I needed them or not," she says, "my parents always find a way to ruin things." Further discussion reveals that Melissa went shopping after a boy who she was interested in did not text her back right away. Concerned, you comment on the possible link between her spending and these text exchanges. She dismisses the idea, however, saying "What's wrong with a little shopping therapy? My sponsor suggested it, now that I'm not relying on smoking anymore!"

Choice Point 4

What would you do about Melissa's excessive spending?

1. Tell her to return the shoes as a way to repair her relationship with her parents.
2. Explore what is helpful and what is unhelpful about her shopping sprees.
3. Request a meeting with the sponsor to discuss the problem her suggestion caused.
4. Stand firm in expressing your concern that her spending may be a symptom of her BPD.
5. Ask about Melissa's reaction to not receiving a text back from her romantic interest, and draw her attention to the interpersonal context (rejection) in which she developed her urge to shop.

Discussion

Melissa has reduced her dependence on marijuana yet still struggles with interpersonal sensitivity, now leading to impulsive spending. The main focus of treatment at this point would be to help Melissa put words to her emotional experience and thereby contain her urges to spend excessively. In that light, prioritizing a discussion of family relationships and of what to do with the shoes is off-target. Similarly, even if Melissa's sponsor did suggest shopping, it will be more effective for now to intervene with Melissa directly than with a third party.

Motivational interviewing techniques are nonjudgmental and hence are a promising technique for with patients with BPD [4]. Asking Melissa what is helpful about shopping will likely be experienced as empathic or validating, reducing her defensiveness. Questions about what is unhelpful, following an empathic inquiry, put Melissa in position to be able to generate alternate perspectives on her actions, something she struggles with while angry at her parents.

A second approach is to stand firm in your concern about her spending. She has already dismissed your first attempt to frame her spending as related to her BPD, probably because she is too emotional to see things from your perspective. To voice that concern effectively you will want to understand, in the same conversation, what specific emotional impact the spending has had. As Melissa herself says, the shopping is therapeutic. You need not question that, but merely get her to consider spending lesser amounts. If you focus on the emotions that drive Melissa to spend, she can calm down, returning her to a state of mind in which she can devise a better coping strategy.

A third approach is to rewind, before the shopping, to help her elaborate her frame of mind during her text message exchange with this romantic interest. Starting there, you can ask how her emotions, thoughts, and urges unfolded. It would not be surprising if you heard that the idea to buy expensive shoes came not from the sponsor, but arose when Melissa called her sponsor and the sponsor did not pick up the phone.

Answers

1. U
2. H
3. U
4. P
5. H

Principles and Clinical Pearls

1. When a patient with BPD manages to control one problematic or impulsive behavior, another one often crops up. Patients often need your help to grasp that new behaviors are driven by the same emotional sensitivities as old ones.
2. When patients engage in behavior that is obviously maladaptive, or "point the finger" at third parties, it is easy for the therapy to get bogged down in insisting on one's own point of view, or misdirecting interventions at people other than the patient. Keep in mind that patients' own emotional responses and judgments are the primary changeable cause of their difficulties, so should be targeted as the ultimate locus of change.
3. When patients are angry and defensive, they are least able to see other points of view. There may be times when it is important to maintain your position, but to be effective you must pair expression of your own stance with efforts to see and connect with the patient's distress.

Case Continues...

Melissa's marijuana use and spending gradually fall. She reports better mood, memory, and motivation. She returns to swimming after a break of 4 or 5 years. Then, one session she comes in sobbing. Her birthday was just a few days ago, and you wonder what has her so upset. She tells you, "They didn't call me! None of them! No calls, no texts, nothing!" Confused, you ask who she is talking about. "My friends! The ones I used to get high with. They know it was my birthday, but they didn't say anything!" Without waiting for you to comment, she adds "It makes me feel so worthless. Then yesterday one of them texted to see if I wanted to smoke up with her and I couldn't say no." She continues, "I know this is my BPD, but I really needed to see someone, even if that meant getting high. The other girls I've been hanging out with recently didn't even know it was my birthday, we're not that close yet. My parents told me not to be so dramatic and I know they're right, but I just can't help it." She looks at you and asks if you agree with her parents that she is overreacting again.

Choice Point 5

How would you respond to Melissa's emotions about her birthday?

1. Encourage her not to be upset, because she is much better off without her old friends.
2. Role-play with her in session around how to set healthy, respectful boundaries with old friends.
3. Suggest that she ignore her parents, as they obviously do not understand her.
4. Praise her for recognizing on her own that this interpersonal shift is a trigger.
5. Empathize with the loss of meaningful friendships, no matter how problematic her behavior afterward.

Discussion

Melissa has clearly progressed in treatment. Her functioning has improved. She uses marijuana less and thinks more clearly. Her underlying interpersonal sensitivity remains, yet now she recognizes what triggers it. That awareness has allowed her to take a mental step back to consider alternative viewpoints.

You may indeed think that Melissa is better off away from the influence of a substance-using peer group. Nevertheless, her distress at feeling more alone is understandable. Suggesting she push aside those feelings will therefore be invalidating. Role-playing around setting limits is a helpful concrete intervention – though it may be premature. You would want to be careful first to validate Melissa's emotions.

As for answering Melissa's question about whether you agree with her parents that she overreacted, the key is to answer in a way that stimulates her own reflection about the problem. In the "heat of the moment" when patients demand an immediate response to such questions, clinicians often collapse reactively into either wholly accepting or wholly contradicting patients' point of view. Neither stance is productive, ultimately, because black-or-white agreement or disagreement fails to model or stimulate curiosity about how patients arrive at their own points of view. The scenario described above makes it sounds like Melissa's parents do understand her vulnerability, though they came across in a dismissive way. Rather than takes sides on whose point of view is "correct," you can be more effective by helping her explore how her parents might have arrived at such a conclusion, and how she arrives at her own (likely ambivalent) conclusion, without offering your own judgments as the arbiters of reality. Regardless of any other action you take, praising her achievement of recognizing a trigger is advisable. Lastly, it is important to recognize that, credit card drama aside, Melissa sounds upset about her loss of close friendships. Her achievement of sobriety leaves her trapped by a choice between new friends who do not know it's her birthday and old friends who will lead her astray. Empathy for her dilemma and for the relationship loss provides needed validation during a predictably difficult transition.

Answers

1. U
2. P
3. U
4. H
5. H

Principles and Clinical Pearls

1. People with BPD will have difficulty seeing things from other people's point of view when upset, so intervention in any situation usually starts with empathy.
2. When patients with BPD ask a direct question, a direct answer is often appropriate. Whether you answer a question or not, explaining your choice allows you to model for the patient how her or his actions have an impact on your mind.
3. Effective treatment for BPD results in people having: (1) less extreme emotions in reaction to interpersonal triggers; (2) more recognition of the links between triggers and emotions; and (3) a greater ability to make sense of the situation by putting it into words rather than into actions.

Summary of Clinical Approach

This case illustrates key principles of treating patients with borderline personality disorder (BPD) and comorbid substance use. Chief among these is to consider whether substance use occurs within the BPD framework of interpersonal hypersensitivity. Patients who meet the diagnostic threshold for an independent substance use disorder may require concurrent substance treatment. Effective techniques to address substance use, such as motivational interviewing and referral to 12-step programs, can readily be integrated into treatment for BPD. Sustained sobriety, or engagement in substance treatment, are not prerequisites for participation in treatment for BPD, but are often necessary to its success. Another key principle is to ensure that treatment is guided by the patient's goals and values. This will maximize initial motivation and, if motivation wanes, knowing the patient's goals and values gives the therapist a ready-made intervention. A further key principle is that you can expect risky or reckless behaviors, once treated, to resurface in different forms, until the underlying interpersonal hypersensitivity is better managed.

Clinician Experience: Wish to Feel Helpful by Increasing Intersession Availability
Watching a person who engages in behaviors, including drug and alcohol misuse, which are harmful and interferes with their treatment can be a challenge for providers. Some may react with "leaning back" by adopting a blandly

supportive stance that avoids the real issues. Others may become overly critical or punitive, and fail to connect with the fact that the patient is likely also
concerned about the substance misuse. The sweet spot, of course, involves
naming the substance use disorder as a primary treatment issue and attempting to understand how BPD symptoms and the substance use disorder likely
fuel each other in both directions. However, when substance use disorders
become severe, it may become impossible to conduct meaningful BPD treatment, requiring an initial primary focus on substance use disorder treatment to
achieve sobriety. Awareness of role of the clinician's internal experiences in
how the use disorder is addressed can help guard against an unusually fertile
landscape for countertransference enactments.

References

1. Lee NK, Cameron J, Jenner L. A systematic review of interventions for co-occurring substance
   use and borderline personality disorders. Drug Alcohol Rev. 2015;34(6):663–72.
2. Lana F, Sánchez-Gil C, Adroher ND, Pérez V, Feixas G, Martí-Bonany J, Torrens
   M. Comparison of treatment outcomes in severe personality disorder patients with or without
   substance use disorders: a 36-month prospective pragmatic follow-up study. Neuropsychiatr
   Dis Treat. 2016;12:1477–87.
3. Gunderson JG, Links P. Handbook of good psychiatric management for borderline personality
   disorder. Arlington: American Psychiatric Association Publishing; 2014.
4. McMurran M, Cox WM, Whitham D, Hedges L. The addition of a goal-based motivational
   interview to treatment as usual to enhance engagement and reduce dropouts in a personality
   disorder treatment service: results of a feasibility study for a randomized controlled trial. Trials.
   2013;14:50.

Dr. Fleisher graduated from Harvard Medical School. He completed residency in adult psychia-
try and fellowship in child and adolescent psychiatry at the University of California, Los Angeles
(UCLA) Health System. Currently, he serves as an Assistant Clinical Professor of Psychiatry at
UCLA and maintains a private practice in Beverly Hills. He is certified as a supervisor for
Mentalization-Based Treatment for borderline personality disorder, specializing in work with ado-
lescents and families. He is also a trainer for Good Psychiatric Management of Borderline
Personality Disorder.

Medical Comorbidities

10

Claire Brickell

Choice Point Index
1. Making the connection between medical problems and emotional symptoms in BPD.
2. Making initial changes to promote physical health and gain mastery.
3. Managing an acute physical symptom.
4. Maintaining the treatment alliance and coordinating with medical providers.
5. Setting expectations for longer term treatment.

Case Introduction

Maria is a 47-year-old woman who is referred to you for psychopharmacology by her primary care physician (PCP). She has multiple medical problems including asthma, obesity, fibromyalgia, and migraine headaches. She has been to the emergency room three times in the past month seeking rescue medication for intense headaches. Each time, she has received intravenous pain medication. She is also diagnosed with depression, and describes near-constant anxiety that prevents her from sleeping well at night. Her PCP was concerned by her escalating use of benzodiazepines (now lorazepam 1 mg three times daily), but nothing else seems to help her anxiety. He is both frustrated by and worried about Maria, who does not do a good job of taking care of her asthma, and continues to smoke a pack of cigarettes daily despite multiple efforts to quit.

C. Brickell, M.D.
McLean Hospital and Harvard Medical School, Belmont, MA, USA
e-mail: cbrickell@partners.org

© Springer International Publishing AG, part of Springer Nature 2018
B. Palmer, B. Unruh (eds.), *Borderline Personality Disorder*,
https://doi.org/10.1007/978-3-319-90743-7_10

When you first meet Maria, she appears physically unwell. She is obese, walks with difficulty, and has an intermittent cough. She has a litany of complaints, including how hard it was to get to your office and how her niece was late picking her up. At the same time, you are impressed by her wicked sense of humor and her obvious intelligence.

Maria has been suffering from depression since she was a teenager, and has taken various medications without much benefit. They seem to work for a while but then peter out. Her weight began to spiral out of control when she was in college and began binge-eating to handle the stress of exams. Sometimes she also eats to manage more chronic feelings of being "bored" or "empty." She has a remote history of cutting herself and had one suicide attempt shortly after college graduation, when a long-time boyfriend broke up with her. Although she did well in college, she has since bounced from job to job, and has been on disability for the past 7 years because of her asthma. She has a large extended family and relies on a series of nieces and nephews to help her with her medical appointments. She describes constantly being on the outs with someone in her family, and worries that they are "getting sick of me."

Maria is wondering what you can do to help her feel better. She would like to try a different medication regimen that would be more helpful for her mood, anxiety, and headaches.

Choice Point 1

For each intervention, choose H: "helpful," U: "unhelpful or harmful," or P: "perhaps helpful, with reservations."

With regard to Maria's request for medication, do you:

1. Add gabapentin to her medication regimen because it is less addictive than lorazepam and may also be helpful for fibromyalgia.
2. Tell her that she is not likely to feel better until she quits smoking and gets better control over her asthma.
3. Make the diagnosis of borderline personality disorder.
4. Obtain additional history from her PCP and family.

Discussion

Maria is at much greater risk due to medical complications (e.g., asthma attack, heart disease) than she is from suicide or self-injury. She is herself primarily focused on her "biological" symptoms. Nevertheless, she does meet criteria for borderline personality disorder. As is typical for middle-aged adults with BPD, her more flagrant self-destructive symptoms (e.g., cutting, suicidality) have diminished, but she continues to struggle with interpersonal hypersensitivity and remains functionally incapacitated by her disorder.

BPD is best conceptualized as an "engine" that fuels symptoms in many other domains, including medical and physical illness. Studies show increased association between BPD and diverse medical conditions including chronic fatigue, fibromyalgia, TMJ syndrome, back pain, diabetes, hypertension, obesity, osteoarthritis, and urinary incontinence [4]; stroke and ischemic heart disease [6]; arteriosclerosis, cardiovascular disease, gastrointestinal disease, hypertension, liver disease, venereal disease, and "any assessed medical condition"[3]. BPD can also confer decreased responsiveness to standard medical treatment for conditions such as migraines [7]. At the level of medical service utilization, BPD is associated with increased medical office visits[1, 8], medication prescriptions[8, 9], emergency room visits[2], use of higher numbers of primary care physicians and medical specialists[10], telephone calls to medical offices[9], and inpatient hospitalizations[2].

Given these associations, BPD likely affects not only Maria's anxiety but also the ways she experiences and seeks treatment for pain and medical symptoms. For example, people with BPD often feel quite poorly about themselves and lack a sense of being able to capably manage in the world. This sense of hopelessness, coupled with the need for immediate relief from intolerable feelings of sadness, anger, or guilt, can lead to self-destructive behavior. Maria has not cut herself in many years, but she continues to damage her body through overeating, smoking, and poor compliance with her asthma medication. Seen through the lens of BPD, her trips to the emergency room can be seen as not only an attempt to get rid of her headache, but also an opportunity to have her suffering concretely acknowledged and managed within a world she otherwise perceives as uncaring and unhelpful.

Although gabapentin is perhaps less harmful than lorazepam, adding another medication at this juncture is beside the point, and only reinforces the idea that she needs to seek relief from medication. It is true that quitting smoking and managing her asthma will help her feel better, but she first needs to understand the relationship between her physical health and her emotional symptoms. Obtaining additional information is not harmful, and learning more about "failed" medical treatments may build a more persuasive case for rethinking her approach in light of a new BPD diagnosis. However, you already have enough information to make and share the BPD diagnosis.

Answers

1. U
2. P
3. H
4. H

Principles and Clinical Pearls

1. Patients with BPD are at increased risk for a wide variety of medical problems. They are high utilizers of medical (as well as psychiatric) services, but tend to respond more poorly than most to treatment.
2. There are strong ties between emotional symptoms and physical health. For example, medical problems can be a result of poor self-care or overtly self-destructive behavior. Medical care can also gratify the need to be taken care of, or to have suffering concrete acknowledged.
3. Making any medication change before discussing the diagnosis of BPD and the relationship between physical and emotional symptoms runs the risk of erroneously reinforcing the belief that medication is the way to seek relief.

Choice Point 2

Priorities in Maria's treatment include:

1. Tapering off lorazepam.
2. Smoking cessation.
3. Finding meaningful activity.
4. Referral to a DBT group.

Discussion

Tapering off benzodiazepines is a worthwhile though challenging treatment goal for many BPD patients. Safely discontinuing them, especially in an outpatient with medical comorbidity, means decreasing the dose only gradually. Benzodiazepine tapers are ideally initiated with patients' buy-in, although this is not necessary when the risks of maintaining the prescription outweigh the benefits. You can facilitate increased collaboration around tapering by providing education around why high benzodiazepine doses are dangerous, including risks of worsening behavioral disinhibition (leading to more impulsive, more lethal self-harming and suicidal behavior). An additional risk for BPD patients attempting more ambitious psychological treatments is that benzodiazepines can impair emotional exposure and re-experiencing processes that are essential for deeper personality change. Prior to beginning the taper, you should help patients develop a plan for how else to manage anxiety. This plan will likely be multifactorial, including matching behavioral skills with known triggers, developing more rapport and trust with you, and possibly time-limited use of alternative safer anxiolytics while the taper is ongoing.

Quitting smoking is one of the most important things that Maria can do for her medical and psychological health. It also provides her with an opportunity to gain mastery and reach an achievable goal, serving as a counterpoint to chronic low self-esteem and feelings of incapacity. BPD patients should be enlisted as active participants by collaboratively setting a quit date, considering biological aides such as bupropion and nicotine replacement therapies, and making a plan in advance to help deal with cravings and triggers.

Functional impairment is one of the most persistent symptoms of BPD, and social rehabilitation should be a core objective of any treatment approach. Boredom, feelings of worthlessness, loneliness, and frustration are all contributing to Maria's physical and psychological stress. Cultivating structured and meaningful activities should be a priority, if not a condition, of her ongoing treatment with you.

A DBT group would likely be helpful for Maria, providing both a way to learn skillful behavior and a source of social connection with peers. However, such resources are not readily available in all practice settings. You and she should not wait for a DBT group to expect her to begin making progress.

Answers

1. H
2. H
3. H
4. P

Principles and Clinical Pearls

1. People with BPD are more likely to successfully make changes to promote their health when they have meaningful structure and the opportunity to gain mastery over their lives.
2. Help patients decrease their reliance on harmful substances, including benzodiazepines and tobacco. Where possible, enlist them as active participants in the quitting process.

Case Continues...

Maria resists your suggestion that she find a volunteer position, stating that she gets tired too easily, her back hurts, and that she is anxious around new people. She tearfully accuses you of "judging me because I am fat" and of treating her like she is "just making everything up." She becomes dismissive of the BPD diagnosis, insisting that her headaches are her main problem, and that she would feel better and be more able to take care of herself if only she could get them under control. She cannot believe that you would treat her in this "callous and insensitive" way, despite your acknowledgement of her suffering.

Choice Point 3

Regarding Maria's emphasis on her headaches, do you:

1. Tell her that migraines are psychosomatic and they will disappear when she achieves psychiatric stability.
2. Prescribe her a medication, such as amitriptyline or topiramate, to prevent headaches.
3. Teach her some distress tolerance skills so that she can better manage the pain the next time she gets a migraine.
4. Ask her to keep a detailed record of when she gets headaches, what triggers them, and what relationship they have to interpersonal stress.

Discussion

You do not have enough information to say with certainty that Maria's headaches "aren't real," and doing so is likely to be perceived as cruel. You should, however, educate her on the relationship between stress and pain and the fact that people with BPD are more sensitive to pain and less able to manage it well. You can offer to help her come up with a plan to better cope with her pain.

Prescribing medications to lessen headaches is outside of your area of expertise, and colludes with the idea that her main problem is pain and can be solved with medication. You should, however, coordinate with her PCP to make sure that she is receiving standard-of-care treatment for her headaches.

Teaching Maria distress tolerance skills may help her better manage the pain of migraines, but should be preceded by some more education about the relationship between BPD and general health to increase her motivation and commitment to the harder path of managing migraines behaviorally (not purely pharmacologically) and taking a multifaceted approach to improve her general health.

Having her keep a detailed record of the onset of headaches, associated triggers, and their relatedness to interpersonal stress is a way of proceeding thoughtfully that also teaches Maria the solution begins with her becoming an accountable, active participant in her treatment. It is an opportunity to highlight the relationship between medical and psychological symptoms, without dismissing her headaches as "not real."

Answers

1. U
2. U
3. P
4. H

Principles and Clinical Pearls

1. Do not get into a debate with patients about whether or not their symptoms are "real." Instead, provide education regarding the relationship between physical and emotional pain. This provides the rationale for including psychological interventions as part of a multifaceted approach to managing illness.
2. Know the limits of your knowledge and your practice, and do not get involved in managing medical conditions outside of your expertise. Do communicate regularly with primary care physicians or other specialists who are expert in the relevant treatment.
3. Challenge patients' passivity in relation to the medical system by enlisting them as active participants (e.g., in tracking symptoms or evaluating treatment response). Encourage ongoing attention to the interplay between psychological and physical factors.

Case Continues...

Over the next few months, Maria's attendance is increasingly inconsistent. She misses an appointment because she was "too sick" and another because she was in the emergency room. Her PCP calls you to say that she has been making frequent appointments and comes in with nonspecific complaints of pain or insomnia. He is wondering why she is not coming to your appointments yet coming so frequently to his.

Choice Point 4

With regard to Maria's pattern of attending medical and psychiatric appointments, you should:

1. Tell her that she is meeting with her PCP too often and that this is an inappropriate use of resources.
2. Wonder with her whether there is something about your sessions together that makes it hard for her to come in.
3. Frame her visits to her PCP as a way to get attention and caring.
4. Renew your efforts to enlist her in developing meaningful activities.

Discussion

Choice 1 sounds shaming and punitive, and is unlikely to help Maria reflect on the function her PCP appointments serve. It is also important that you and her PCP demonstrate that you are both on the same team, united in your desire to help her feel and function better. This can be conveyed by arranging a joint meeting with Maria and her PCP either in person or by phone to discuss treatment planning.

Encouraging Maria to consider what makes it hard for her to see you consistently may help improve her relationship with you as well as her reflectiveness about how interpersonal experiences influence her health-related decisions. She may do so less defensively if you acknowledge that you think there is something you are doing that it is making it more comfortable for her to see her PCP. You know you are being challenging by asking her to change her usual ways of coping with distress, so you can suggest this as a possible contributing factor.

Your formulation of the interpersonal and emotional function of Maria's visits to her PCP may be accurate. But, its utility to her depends on how you present your understanding of an aspect of her functioning that she may not see within herself. It may help to invoke a universal human need for attention and caring, which you believe she deserves like anyone else. It may also help to remind her that individuals with BPD have heightened needs for empathy and support because they generally grew up feeling deprived of them. Maria will be helped tremendously if you help her make the connection between her visits to her PCP and these heightened inter-personal and emotional needs.

Renewing your efforts to enlist Maria in developing life-giving nontreatment activities may seem counterintuitive, especially since previously she has expressed reluctance and your determination to reverse her disability has generated friction in your relationship. However, having a sense of connection within a community and being able to contribute meaningfully to the world around her will help her reduce her need for PCP and emergency room visits.

Answers

1. U
2. H
3. P
4. H

Principles and Clinical Pearls

1. Maintaining an alliance with a patient with BPD and somatic complaints is difficult, particularly if you are challenging the patient's view of their core problem. Be prepared to acknowledge that what you are asking of the patient (i.e., changing usual ways of managing distress) is painful and difficult.
2. Do not shame patients for needing attention and caring. Validate their heightened emotional and interpersonal needs, even if you are concerned that they are meeting them inappropriately through medical intervention.
3. Do not set up medical and psychiatric care as mutually exclusive alternatives to one other. Instead, emphasize the synergy between good physical and good men-

tal health. Be openly collaborative with medical providers to demonstrate that you are part of the same team.

Case Continues...

Together, you and Maria continue to weather a variety of medical crises. She begrudgingly tells you that she appreciates you sticking with her, even though she can sometimes be "a pain in the butt." You and her PCP agree that she should have regular, scheduled appointments with him so that she can count on being seen without having to be sick to justify these visits. She is aware that the two of you are in regular communication about her treatment goals, around which she feels increasingly aligned with you. She has joined a weekly book club and has started going to church regularly. Her ER and PCP visits gradually lessen.

Choice Point 5

With regard to Maria's progress, you should:

1. Tell her that she is doing much better and can return to working only with her PCP.
2. Enlist her in setting additional goals and priorities.
3. Expect that treatment will be easier from now on.

Discussion

For a patient with somatic symptoms such as Maria's, you should expect progress to be slow. It is hard work to shift away from a "medical model" of illness. Maria is used to seeking care and attention from medical doctors and it is challenging for her to learn to rely more on herself and less on them. At the same time, you are working to help her put more emphasis on prevention (e.g., smoking cessation, good asthma care), which all people find difficult to sustain. Your work is still cut out for you, although having a solid framework will help your work get easier.

Recovery from BPD is in and of itself a worthy medical goal associated with reduction in chronic medical conditions; poor health-related lifestyle choices such as higher pack-per-day smoking, daily sleep medication use, overuse of pain medications, and exercise deficit; utilization of costly medical services such as medical ER visits, medical hospitalizations, and radiological studies; and less incidents of quitting or losing a job due to medical reasons [5]. Your ongoing involvement in Maria's care can help her continue to progress in the many areas where her psychiatric disorder and medical problems remain inextricably linked.

Answers

1. U
2. H
3. P

Principles and Clinical Pearls

1. Expect slow and painstaking progress with patients with BPD and multiple medical problems.
2. Maintain a consistent and steady focus on rehabilitation and recovery.
3. Recovery from BPD is associated with an improvement in physical symptoms, decreased medical risk, and lower use of medical services.

Summary of Clinical Approach

Your goal as a psychopharmacologist for patients with BPD and medical comorbidities such as Maria's is to help make the link between physical symptoms, need for relief and caretaking, and interpersonal and emotional difficulties at the core of BPD. Helping her understand the psychological drivers of her pain and her poor self-care is a critical element in structuring her treatment and your role within it. She comes to you as a passive victim of circumstance, asking for more help with "getting rid of the pain." You work toward that goal by helping her become more active, more accountable, and more engaged in building a richer life for herself outside of being a chronic medical patient. At the same time, it is unrealistic to expect that her physical ailments will completely dissipate, or that she will easily be able to improve her management of them. Steady attention, repetition, and close coordination with her PCP are all important elements in your treatment.

> **Clinician Experience: Intolerance of Suffering**
> Many of us became clinicians because we want to help people. It can therefore feel terrible to face a patient who is suffering and begging for help. It feels even more counterintuitive (and even cruel) to withhold the thing that they are asking for (e.g., pain medication). However, this good-intentioned attitude can be extremely harmful for patients with BPD. They can end up taking high doses of multiple medications, relying too heavily on somatic treatments, and losing or never building their own sense of agency. It can be helpful to remind the patient—and yourself—that the best form of caring is one that is effective in helping her build a better life. Saying "no" can be an act of caring, and shows that you value the patient enough to stick to your guns and provide the best possible clinical care, underscoring their capacity to live up to their own best interests.

References

1. Ansell EB, Sanislow CA, McGlashan TH, Grilo CM. Psychosocial impairment and treatment utilization by patients with borderline personality disorder, other personality disorders, mood and anxiety disorders, and a healthy comparison group. Compr Psychiatry. 2007;48:329–36.
2. Black DW, Blum N, Letuchy E, Carney Doebbeling C, Forman-Hoffman VL, Doebbeling BN. Borderline personality disorder and traits in veterans: psychiatric comorbidity, healthcare utilization, and quality of life along a continuum of severity. CNS Spectr. 2006;11:680e9.
3. El-Gabalawy R, Katz LY, Sareen J. Comorbidity and associated severity of borderline personality disorder and physical health conditions in a nationally representative sample. Psychosom Med. 2010;72:641–7.
4. Frankenburg FR, Zanarini MC. The association between borderline personality disorder and chronic medical illnesses, poor health-related lifestyle choices, and costly forms of health care utilization. J Clin Psychiatry. 2004;65(12):1660–5.
5. Keuroghlian AS, Frankenburg FR, Zanarini MC. The relationship of chronic medical illnesses, poor health-related lifestyle choices, and health care utilization to recovery status in borderline patients over a decade of prospective follow-up. J Psychiatr Res. 2013;47(10):1499–506.
6. Moran P, Stewart R, Brugha T, Bebbington P, Bhugra D, Jenkins R, Coid JW. Personality disorder and cardiovascular disease: results from a national household survey. J Clin Psychiatry. 2007;68(1):69–74.
7. Rothrock J, Lopez I, Zweilfer R, Andress-Rothrock D, Drinkard R, Walters N. Borderline personality disorder and migraine. Headache. 2007;47(1):22–6.
8. Sansone RA, Sansone LA, Wiederman MW. Borderline personality disorder and health care utilization in a primary care setting. South Med J. 1996;89:1162–5.
9. Sansone RA, Wiederman MW, Sansone LA. Borderline personality symptomatology, experience of multiple types of trauma, and health care utilization among women in a primary care setting. J Clin Psychiatry. 1998;59:108–11.
10. Sansone RA, Farukhi S, Wiederman MW. Utilization of primary care physicians in borderline personality. Gen Hosp Psychiatry. 2011;33:343–6.

Dr. Brickell is a child and adolescent psychiatrist on staff at the Gunderson Residence of McLean Hospital, an intensive residential treatment program for women with severe personality disorders. She is a graduate of Harvard Medical School and completed residency and fellowship training at Massachusetts General and McLean Hospital. She is committed to improving personality disorder treatment, particularly through teaching medical students and psychiatry residents.

Psychiatric Comorbidities and Appropriate Psychopharmacology

James A. Jenkins

Choice Point Index
1. Considering personality disorder diagnoses in referred patients
2. Avoiding reactive prescribing by focusing on effective psychosocial interventions
3. Understanding the evidence for medications in BPD
4. Applying a principled approach to medications in an ongoing treatment

Case Introduction

Julie is a 24-year-old woman who comes to the hospital's outpatient clinic for an intake appointment with a resident psychiatrist as part of her discharge plan from her fourth admission to the hospital's mood disorders unit. Julie's most recent hospitalization, one month prior to the intake appointment, was after a suicide attempt by overdose on diphenhydramine. This was her third suicide attempt by overdose within the past two years, none of which required medical intervention. Given Julie's history of numerous failed medication trials, Julie's hospital course included eight treatments of right unilateral electroconvulsive therapy (ECT). ECT was described as "modestly effective" at reducing her depressive symptoms and ruminations about suicide. After discharge, she was referred to continue weekly outpatient ECT with the hope that she would continue to benefit from the treatment. Her discharge paperwork included diagnoses of atypical bipolar disorder, panic disorder without agoraphobia, post-traumatic stress disorder, and attention deficit disorder. In addition, she has medical diagnoses that include migraines and obesity. Her

J. A. Jenkins, M.D.
Harvard Medical School, McLean Hospital, Belmont, MA, USA
e-mail: jajenkins@partners.org

© Springer International Publishing AG, part of Springer Nature 2018
B. Palmer, B. Unruh (eds.), *Borderline Personality Disorder*,
https://doi.org/10.1007/978-3-319-90743-7_11

discharge summary alludes to several contentious family meetings during her hospitalization, which punctuated an otherwise pleasant and fully cooperative stay. When the resident gets his schedule for the day, he notices that Julie's listed chief complaint for the visit is, "I want to quit ECT."

Choice Point 1

For each choice point, choose H: "helpful," U: "unhelpful or harmful," or P: "perhaps helpful, with reservations."

Given the referral information and discharge summary, how should the resident physician structure his intake appointment?

1. Frame the intake appointment as an opportunity to learn about each other and give anticipatory guidance that changes to the treatment plan, both medications and ECT, will be considered only after a treatment agreement is reached.
2. Accept the diagnoses on the discharge summary that the attending psychiatrist with expertise in mood disorders gave Julie. Expect to continue the treatment plan that was recommended on discharge and focus on updates in neurovegetative symptoms since discharge.
3. When possible during the intake, emphasize the severe nature of the patient's bipolar diagnosis and use motivational interviewing techniques to encourage her to continue with ECT as previously arranged.
4. Allow Julie to speak with minimal interruptions about her experience with her illness, hospitalizations, and current ideas about what would be most helpful for her.
5. During the intake appointment, budget adequate time to take a thorough social history, occupational history, and inventory of past and current relationships.

Discussion

There is enough information prior to the intake appointment to raise suspicion that Julie may have a comorbid personality disorder diagnosis. Her multiple suicide attempts, frequent hospitalizations, the atypical nature of her mood disorder, lack of response to prior therapeutics, and allusions to interpersonal difficulties should lead the new psychiatrist to broaden the differential diagnosis to include the possibility of a personality disorder. Good psychiatric care requires that clinicians avoid the heuristic biases that all physicians are susceptible to: most notably the anchoring bias and confirmation bias. The anchoring bias is a tendency to accept initial diagnosis without further thought, and the confirmation bias is selectively attending to pieces of information that confirm one's first impression [1]. When seeing a patient for the first time, it is both helpful to know what others (including more senior clinicians) have thought while also keeping an open mind for new information or observations that might be more apparent in a different context. Patients with personality disorder pathology are especially susceptible to presenting differently across different environments and interpersonal interactions, which further necessitates careful monitoring of one's cognitive biases.

Including personality disorders on the differential can help clinicians approach initial appointments in a manner which reduces reactive interventions and can set the expectation from the start that the patient is an active agent in her treatment and not the passive recipient of medications. In addition, this can help the clinician to budget his time to focus on Julie's social history more than he might in other intake appointments. For someone with a personality disorder, the social history is likely to reveal unstable relationships, mismatches in education and occupational functioning, evidence of risky and impulsive behaviors, difficulties knowing and carrying out one's own goals and values, and problems with substance abuse. Knowledge of these factors is essential to make the personality disorder diagnosis and to appropriately assess suicide risk.

Placing too much importance on ECT or the bipolar diagnosis is likely to diminish the patient's sense of agency, decrease curiosity and self-reflection about one's contributions to the difficulties in her life, lead to further externalizing behaviors, and, paradoxically, lead the patient to feel invalidated that her complex problems could be solved by simple interventions. For those with a primary personality disorder diagnosis, clinicians' unambiguous assertions about the helpfulness of psychotropics and neurotherapeutics can stimulate feelings of hopelessness and futility if these interventions fail to provide relief from their symptoms. That being said, there is a 15% comorbidity between BPD and bipolar disorder, therefore maintaining even attention to all of the patient's symptoms is necessary.

Answers

1. H
2. U
3. U
4. P
5. H

Clinical Pearls

1. Clinicians should be aware that patients with personality disorders may present differently in different contexts, and the diagnosis of a personality disorder should be on the differential for patients with recurring suicidality and significant interpersonal or occupational dysfunction that cannot be adequately accounted for by a more classical affective episode (i.e., mania) or psychiatric diagnosis (i.e., schizophrenia).
2. It is crucial to be nonreactive in prescribing medications or changing treatment plans in patients with personality disorders.
3. Patients with a personality disorder should be encouraged to take an active role as a collaborator in their treatment.

4. Clinicians should aim to avoid a dichotomous stance regarding the helpfulness or lack of potential benefit that medications and neurotherapeutics can provide at reducing symptoms.

Case Continues...

Julie arrives to her appointment ten minutes late and without the requested paperwork that was sent to her prior to her appointment. During the intake, she is in tears and has markedly increased rate of speech with a linear thought process. She states that her boyfriend was unfaithful toward her while she was in the hospital and that she worries that he will soon leave her. Just prior to her appointment, she saw him texting on his mobile phone and was suspicious that he was texting another woman. She responded to this by taking his phone and destroying it in the garbage disposal, a decision she now regrets. She continues to have suicidal thoughts, but no urges to act on these thoughts, and discloses to the resident psychiatrist that she has been binge drinking and cutting her upper thighs to cope with alternating between "feeling totally overwhelmed and dead inside." She believes that ECT has made her symptoms worse and is now frequently having episodes where she feels "very disconnected from my body, like I am watching things happen to me through fog." She requests an increase in her dose of alprazolam and quetiapine stating that these two medications are "the only things that make me feel even a little better." Review of her medication regimen reveals the following prescriptions: alprazolam 1 mg Q6H PRN anxiety, quetiapine 50 mg TID PRN anxiety and 100 mg at bedtime, dextroamphetamine 10 mg BID, aripiprazole 2.5 mg daily, fluoxetine 60 mg daily, and lithium 900 mg at bedtime.

Choice Point 2

Regarding Julie's request to change her medication regimen, how would you respond?

1. "You are at the maximum recommended dose of alprazolam and I will not be increasing it higher. If you don't agree with this, I would be happy to refer you to a different psychiatrist."
2. "I would like to carefully think about how I can help you so that we don't create more side effects that contribute to your discomfort or make your risk for acting on suicidal thoughts more likely. While I gather more information about your medication history between this visit and our next, are there other things you could do to help decrease the intense sadness and anger that you are feeling?"
3. "We can increase the alprazolam temporarily, but we will have to return back to your current dose within one week. I have some more questions I'd like to get through now as part of the intake."

4. "I am concerned that medications haven't provided you the relief you would like. Maybe we could use this opportunity to see how we might be able to change your approach to your current situation and see if that could reduce your stress. I'd even be willing to see you again next week to see how a change like this works out for you."
5. "These problems require better coping strategies, not medications. Have you thought about going to couple's therapy?"

Discussion

There is more evidence to suggest that Julie likely has a diagnosis of borderline personality disorder (BPD). At this point, she meets all nine of the diagnostic criteria for BPD. The priority of this visit is to establish a working alliance with a patient who is currently in a state of crisis to ensure that she returns for follow-up. Although this is the first meeting with Julie, taking too firm a stance on her medication requests and suggesting that she get care elsewhere would further withdrawal support and could precipitate despair and more overt suicidal behaviors.

Prescribing a medication can have a powerful effect through providing the patient with an external means of self-soothing, when internal means are difficult to generate. The skillful clinician will have to balance remaining nonreactive but thoughtful, expressing concerned attention, validating the patient's distress, and avoiding inadvertently increasing risk with careless prescribing. Although prescribing Julie her requested medications can be alliance building, alliance can also be established by helping her find a solution to a "real-world" problem, being genuine about one's concerns and doubts, and using the therapeutic relationship as a means of reinforcement. Encouraging Julie to find solutions aside from medications and reinforcing it with closer support and more frequent appointments are likely to promote her own self-agency and reduce her overvaluation of medications.

In some situations, short-term prescriptions of medications are necessary to reduce extreme anger, transient psychosis, and worsening impulsivity. If short-term prescriptions are necessary for these symptoms, antipsychotic medications are preferred to benzodiazepines for patients with a BPD diagnosis. There is mounting evidence to suggest that benzodiazepines increase risk of suicide, self-harm, impulsivity, and cognitive impairments in patients with BPD. If Julie persists in requesting an increase in medication and there is further evidence of paranoia and aggression, a temporary increase in quetiapine would be the preferred strategy.

Answers

1. U
2. H
3. U
4. H
5. P

Clinical Pearls

1. It is harmful to withdrawal support and disengage from patients with BPD who are experiencing an interpersonal crisis. This could lead to despair and suicide attempts.
2. Prescribers can offer behavioral interventions, self-soothing skills, and increased frequency of visits to promote skillfulness, agency, and stability rather than passivity and overreliance on medications.
3. Flexibility is essential when treating patients with BPD. Rigidly adhering to the intake format would have been counterproductive in this scenario.
4. If medications are used to reduce aggression, transient psychosis, and impulsivity, then atypical antipsychotics are the preferred treatment and should be used for a limited time, at low doses, and contingent on continued attempts to be more behaviorally skillful and working toward an improved level of functioning.
5. Benzodiazepines are relatively contraindicated in patients with borderline personality disorder.

Case Continues...

Julie agrees to perform a role play in the last several minutes of her appointment to prepare to make an apology to her boyfriend for destroying his mobile phone. She was also able to recall several self-soothing skills she learned on the inpatient unit to comfort herself, and agrees to try these in exchange for another appointment in one week. By the end of the appointment she is no longer anxious and tearful, expresses gratitude for the help received, and states that she looks forward to working with the resident psychiatrist. One week later she returns for follow up and happily reports that her boyfriend was surprised to receive her apology and accepted it. He attributed her willingness to apologize to the ECT, leaving Julie to feel confused as she has not experienced any difference in her symptoms since starting the treatment. She expresses her ongoing confusion about whether ECT is helping her and how this question has made her feel like "I can't trust my own mind." At this appointment, the resident psychiatrist discloses Julie's diagnosis of BPD and provides education about the favorable prognosis and effective treatments that are available. Julie is initially doubtful and rejecting of the resident's diagnosis, questioning how "experts supposedly got the wrong diagnosis, but someone with no experience thinks he knows what's going on with me." The resident validates the difficulty in considering a change in her diagnosis and asks Julie if she would like to review the diagnostic criteria for BPD. In reviewing the criteria, she expressed feeling relief and a sense of being understood. Despite the resident's recommendation that they meet with the ECT team to evaluate the treatment, she decides to forego ongoing ECT. She would like to know what to do about her medications now that her primary diagnosis is BPD.

Choice Point 3

How do you respond to Julie's questions about the use of medications to treat borderline personality disorder?

1. "There are no medications that are approved for the treatment of BPD, nor have any medications shown dramatic benefits."
2. "Medications can be helpful for some of the specific symptoms of BPD and comorbid disorders, but we must be very specific about which symptoms we will target, how to monitor for improvement, and work together to reduce the number of medications and side effects that we expose you to."

Discussion

Although it is true that no medication has been approved for the treatment of BPD, research studies have been complicated by the difficulty assessing for improvement in BPD, fears of violence, worries about suicide, and the high degree of confounding comorbid psychiatric diagnoses in patients with BPD. In general, there are two approaches to the pharmacologic treatment in patients with BPD. One approach is to withdraw all psychotropic medications given the lack of evidence to support their utility. This approach is reflected in the U.K.-based National Institute for Clinical Excellence (NICE) guidelines [2]. A second approach, advocated by the American Psychiatric Association (APA), is to address specific symptom domains within BPD with medications. These domains include affective instability, cognitive perceptual disturbances, and impulsivity and behavioral dyscontrol [3].

In two large meta-analysis [4, 5], there was evidence to suggest modest improvements in the above domains when drugs are targeted in this fashion. In these meta-analyses, mood stabilizers, especially lamotrigine and topiramate, outperformed SSRIs and antipsychotic medications in treating affective instability and behavioral dyscontrol. Antipsychotics primarily have benefits in treating paranoia and transient psychotic symptoms. Additionally, research demonstrates that, with the exception of substance use disorders, anorexia, complex post-traumatic stress disorder (PTSD), and current mania, prioritizing BPD treatment will improve treatment response rates for the comorbid condition.

In Julie's case, the treatment agreement that she and the resident psychiatrist agree on should include a policy that if she fails to respond to a medication, then it will be tapered. The first several sessions should focus on building alliance and, as much as possible, increasing motivation to agree to work toward a slow taper off several of her medications. The resident could offer increased frequency of appointments to support Julie through this process, during which they can focus on working together to build a life outside of treatment.

Answers

1. P
2. H

Clinical Pearls

1. There are no FDA-approved medications for the treatment of BPD. Treatment is based on specific symptom domains. Mood stabilizers may be more helpful for affective instability and impulsivity, whereas antipsychotics may be more helpful for cognitive perceptual disturbances and excessive aggression.
2. Lamotrigine and topiramate have the most current evidence for global improvements in patients with BPD, however this evidence comes from small studies.
3. Treating BPD as the primary disorder may limit the necessity for psychopharmacologic treatment of comorbid diagnoses such as major depressive disorder, panic disorder, and acute post-traumatic stress disorder.

Case Continues...

Julie agrees to a treatment plan that includes conversion of alprazolam to clonazepam 2 mg BID with slow taper (0.25 mg/week) over the course of several weeks. She also agrees to discontinue lithium and fluoxetine given their lack of benefit over the past one year as well as their troublesome side effects of tremor and sexual dysfunction. She agrees to meet weekly with her resident psychiatrist to work on her interpersonal skills, identifying her goals and values, and building day structure. She is reluctant to discontinue her dextroamphetamine because she believes that it helps her to concentrate and is necessary for her to remain awake enough during the day to complete tasks. The resident agrees to continue the dextroamphetamine with the contingency that Julie continues to increase her day structure and find part-time work. The resident also requests that Julie agrees to a planned vacation from the dextroamphetamine for one week after she is off quetiapine, clonazepam, and lithium to reassess its necessity without these sedating medications.

Over the next six months, Julie stops cutting, is no longer suicidal, and started volunteer work at an animal shelter and a part-time job as a barista. She has had no evidence of depression, hypomania, or mania with the medication changes. Two attempts were made to discontinue aripiprazole, but with reduction of dose, Julie's angry outbursts and suspiciousness became more difficult to contain and nearly resulted in loss of her job.

Her medication regimen now includes aripiprazole 10 mg daily and dextroamphetamine 10 mg BID. She honors the agreement to complete a one week trial off the dextroamphetamine and finds no difference in cognition or alertness now that her polypharmacy has been reduced. At this point, she reluctantly agrees to discontinue the dextroamphetamine but laments the loss of a medication that could help her to lose the weight she gained while on quetiapine.

Shortly after the visit where her dextroamphetamine is stopped, Julie discloses several interpersonal struggles she has been having with her two female roommates. She feels restless, anxious, and more dysphoric. She is binge drinking and had a relapse of cutting, albeit much less severe than at the start of treatment. She is distraught about "taking steps backwards" in her treatment and wants to know if she can be restarted on the dextroamphetamine "since everything has gone to shit since you stopped it."

Choice Point 4

What would your next steps in treatment be?

1. Start topiramate to address impulsivity, binge drinking, and affective instability.
2. Refer to a dialectical behavioral therapy (DBT) skills group to work on building interpersonal effectiveness skills.
3. Restart the dextroamphetamine.
4. Express concern that she is sabotaging her treatment as a means of manipulating you into prescribing the dextroamphetamine.

Discussion

It is not unusual for patients with BPD to continue to have interpersonal struggles and impaired social functioning after the more severe symptoms of self-harm, suicidality, and substance abuse remit. Julie's belief that dextroamphetamine is necessary for her success and her fears of failure have likely contributed to recurrence of mood instability since its discontinuation. Within this context, she is likely to be more reassurance seeking, fearful of rejection, and revert to behaviors that she previously used to manage her dysregulation.

Julie may benefit from trial of topiramate or lamotrigine to assist her with management of her mood instability and help to preserve her current level of functioning. Topiramate may have the added benefits of being effective at reducing episodes of binge drinking and promoting weight loss in patients on antipsychotic medications. That said, prescribing it reactively as she suggests would undermine the methodical approach that has been stabilizing to her.

Now that Julie's cognition is clearer, and she has more social interactions outside of treatment, she could benefit from a DBT skills group. At this point, she is in a better position to learn and retain the skills. Because of her improved day structure she will also have opportunities to generalize them to her work and friendships. She might also find that being a part of a group affords her the opportunity to be helpful toward others and to feel less stigmatized and alone with her diagnosis.

While it is possible that Julie's recrudescence of symptoms is motivated by her wish to be prescribed amphetamines, expressing this without also holding some degree of uncertainty is unlikely to be helpful. If there is enough evidence to suggest that Julie's worsening of symptoms is related to her displeasure with the discontinuation of the dextroamphetamine, expressing this in a gentle and questioning manner is more likely to be helpful. The clinician could say, for example, "I can't help but notice that since I stopped prescribing the dextroamphetamine that many of your symptoms have gotten worse. I can't seem to explain this as being the effect of stopping the medication and I wonder if your feeling worse might be related to a change in the way that you feel about our work together?"

Answers

1. P
2. P
3. U
4. U

Clinical Pearls

1. Building a life outside of treatment is essential in the recovery from BPD. However, even after months of treatment, social impairments can persist and patients can remain vulnerable to real or perceived rejections.
2. Use of medications can be justified when used to maintain level of functioning when a patient continues to struggle despite significant efforts. Topiramate and lamotrigine have the best evidence as maintenance treatment for the affective instability and impulsivity associated with BPD. The effect sizes of these medications are small, and they should be seen as adjunctive to the psychological work and case management that is the cornerstone of BPD treatment.
3. Skills groups can be helpful for patients with BPD, especially if they have enough structure to practice generalizing those skills.
4. Patients with BPD are often harmed by excessive polypharmacy. Metabolic effects, sedation, and cognitive impairments from polypharmacy are common occurrences in patients with BPD. These side effects worsen self-esteem, feelings of being a failure, and dependency on others.
5. Nonverbal communications should be directly addressed with patients with BPD to help them learn about the effects of their behaviors on others. When these communications are brought up, it is generally more helpful to do so in a curious and hypothetical manner. Patients are more likely and capable to mentalize with this less threatening approach.

Summary of Clinical Approach

This case captures several key principles of prescribing medications to patients with BPD. In general, the clinician should take an approach of "first do no harm." Patients with BPD are susceptible to reactive polypharmacy that leads to serious side effects with only limited therapeutic gains. In the longest running longitudinal study of BPD, 18.6% of patients reported taking four or more psychotropics, and 6.9% of patients were on five or more medications [6]. In addition, clinical improvement has been demonstrated to be inversely related to the number of psychotropics that patients with BPD are prescribed.

When possible, psychotherapy should be prioritized in treatment over medications, especially psychotherapies that are goal oriented, structured, and emphasize building meaningful work, sense of agency, and accountability. If medications are used, then lamotrigine and topiramate have the most evidence and antipsychotics have some effectiveness for short-term use. Benzodiazepines are relatively contraindicated and medications that present high risk in overdose should be prescribed carefully (e.g. antihypertensives, tricyclic antidepressants, and monoamine oxidase inhibitors).

References

1. Croskerry P. The importance of cognitive errors in diagnosis and strategies to minimize them. Acad Med. 2003;78(8):775.
2. National Institute for Clinical Excellence. Borderline personality disorder, treatment and management. London: The British Psychological society and the Royal College of Psychiatrists; 2009. https://www.nice.org.uk/guidance/cg78/chapter/1-Guidance
3. American Psychiatric Association. Practice guideline for the treatment of patients with borderline personality disorder. American Psychiatric Association: American Psychiatric Pub; 2001. http://psychiatryonline.org/pb/assets/raw/sitewide/practice_guidelines/guidelines/bpd.pdf
4. Ingenhoven T, Lafay P, Rinne T, Passchier J, Duivenvoorden H. Effectiveness of pharmacotherapy for severe personality disorders: meta-analyses of randomized controlled trials. J Clin Psychiatry. 2009;71(1):14–25.
5. Mercer D, Douglass AB, Links PS. Meta-analyses of mood stabilizers, antidepressants and antipsychotics in the treatment of borderline personality disorder: effectiveness for depression and anger symptoms. J Personal Disord. 2009;23(2):156–74.
6. Mary C. Zanarini, Frances R. Frankenburg, John Hennen, Kenneth R. Silk, Mental Health Service Utilization by Borderline Personality Disorder Patients and Axis II Comparison Subjects Followed Prospectively for 6 Years. The Journal of Clin Psychiatry. 2004;65(1):28–36.

James A. Jenkins completed his psychiatry residency at Massachusetts General and McLean Hospital gaining expertise in a variety of evidence-based psychotherapies and milieu treatments for people with complex psychiatric presentations and cooccurring personality disorders. His advanced training includes certification and expert supervision in Dialectical Behavior Therapy, Mentalization-Based Therapy, and Good Psychiatric Management. Dr. Jenkins is interested in the integration of medication management, milieu treatment, and evidence-based psychotherapies to provide the most comprehensive treatment for those whom prior treatments have failed. He currently works at McLean hospital as medical director of the Cambridge Residence program, a DBT-based residential treatment program for transitional aged youth with borderline personality disorder.

Family Engagement

Maureen Smith

Case Introduction

A colleague, Dr. R, contacts you to request that you work with the parents of a new patient of his, Jane, a 20-year-old college sophomore. Jane has just taken a medical leave from school and has returned to her family home where she lives with her parents, Fred and Irene, and younger brother, Joe.

The relevant history you receive is that Jane had been drinking heavily at college and had a number of traumatic sexual encounters when intoxicated. This was an escalation from her freshman year, which she had successfully completed. Jane had all but stopped attending class and was isolating in her residence hall room. Her roommate, with whom she was not getting along, moved out, alerting the resident advisor to the situation. Jane became more despondent, took an overdose of Tylenol, and then told the advisor who sent Jane to the ER.

Jane was quickly stabilized and hospitalized briefly. Her parents were notified and immediately drove up. They were shocked at Jane's suicide attempt and her overall condition. Jane admitted to them that she had been struggling with depression and anxiety for some time and felt unable to manage school. Jane felt she needed "a rest" and agreed to do therapy. Her parents felt overwhelmed and frightened and helped her pack up. Her new therapist, Dr. R, has diagnosed Jane with depression, anxiety, and borderline personality disorder.

When you first meet the parents alone, they are very emotional, recounting how they were unaware of the depths of Jane's problems. Tearfully they state how they thought Jane was a typical college student, partying in a normal fashion. They weep when describing seeing her in the hospital and struggle with their guilt at not recognizing the depths of her pain. They worry they missed signs she was in trouble and are terrified that she will make another suicide attempt.

M. Smith, LICSW
McLean Hospital, Belmont, MA, USA
e-mail: msmith53@partners.org

© Springer International Publishing AG, part of Springer Nature 2018
B. Palmer, B. Unruh (eds.), *Borderline Personality Disorder*,
https://doi.org/10.1007/978-3-319-90743-7_12

Choice Point 1

For each choice point choose H: "helpful", U: "unhelpful or harmful," or P: "perhaps helpful, with reservations".

When Jane's parents express overwhelming guilt, would you:

1. Tell them it is not helpful to feel guilty as they clearly love their daughter and have done their best.
2. Explore more fully what signs they thought they missed.
3. Recognize that as parents it is not only natural for them to feel guilt, but also essential for them to understand how that guilt can also be a limitation.
4. Ask parents to write out their narrative of Jane's life as a way to understand her current troubles.
5. Point out all the ways Jane has kept them in the dark about her emotional pain.

Discussion

This is a critical time to establish a therapeutic alliance with Jane's parents. It is a good start that they did not present in an overly defensive way ("we did our best; it's not our fault") but were able to be open with their fear, guilt, and sense of responsibility. It is helpful to note that some guilt is healthy and a necessary component of self-reflection and one's moral compass. It is not something to be ignored or absolved from (#1).

It is important to start with the assumption that the parents have done their best, and they can do better. If parents feel you are judgmental, it will threaten their sense of being understood and accepted. Many parents struggle with feeling intimidated and judged negatively by mental health professionals. Focusing at this early stage on what they did wrong (#2) can feel critical and threaten the alliance. As in #3, you want to normalize their effort to be a good parent, including helping them understand what they can learn from their guilt. This will be an opening for you to establish the goals of your work with them: helping parents identify how they may need to change and how to adopt a more effective style of parenting wherein they decrease their reactivity and increase their understanding/recognition of Jane's experience.

Asking parents to write out their narrative of Jane's life (#4) can give you valuable information, not only about her development, but also about how the parents have experienced and "see" their daughter. It should be a suggestion/request, not a demand.

Finally, (#5) it is early to focus on the meanings behind daughter holding her emotional struggles from her parents. You likely do not know enough about the family dynamic. Parents could experience this line of questioning as blaming of their daughter and absolving them of guilt which will surely backfire. In addition, though you want to encourage them to have a more curious stance about their daughter, they may need help avoiding judgment about her perceived motives. Never underestimate the strength and loyalty of the family system. Parents need to see you as an ally of them and their daughter.

Answers

1. U
2. P
3. H
4. H
5. P

Principles and Clinical Pearls

1. Establishing an alliance with parents where they feel valued and welcome as an important component of their adult child's treatment is key.
2. It will be immediately helpful for parents to understand that young adults with BPD require different things from their parents than other people, and for you to predict that appreciating this is going to be a learning curve.
3. Instill, model and practice a nonjudgmental, curious, and collaborative approach with parents. You do not have all the answers.

Case Continues...

After meeting the parents, you set up a time to meet with Jane to get her perspective on her family relationships. She is surprisingly critical of her parents, saying they forced her to attend the college she went to - which was a disaster - and that they are critical and demanding, do not understand her, and have their own serious mental health issues. She sees her younger brother as spoiled and entitled due in large part to her parents' indulgent treatment of him. She believes her parents strongly prefer him to her. She reports that she and brother "hate each other," and he avoids her. You are struck by the different pictures she and her parents present. Gentle questioning of her only provokes a more blaming attitude toward her family. She flatly refuses to attend any sessions with her parents.

For their part, parents are hurt and bewildered at Jane's "transformation" from a high-achieving, seemingly happy (although sensitive and sometimes moody) girl to the angry, withdrawn daughter isolating in her room.

Choice Point 2

As you decide how to proceed with the family work, you:

1. Regret not meeting initially with Jane and her parents together, as then you might have gotten a more coherent picture of the family.
2. Agree with Jane that there seem to be problems in the family, but the only way to address them is to immediately begin family therapy together.

3. Plan a "parallel process" in which Jane's therapy can be complemented by parents working with you to learn about BPD and how to better understand and support Jane's treatment.
4. Tell Jane and her parents that if particularly challenging issues arise, you are open to meeting together with the entire family to problem-solve.
5. Decide that the brother is keeping a healthy distance from Jane, which you will support by not asking that he be part of the family work.

Discussion

Although it is possible that you could have seen less conflict meeting with them together (#1), it is more likely that you could have had an explosive session that might adversely affect the family's perception of such work as helpful. Parents could present a well-defended position that minimized problems silencing and further alienating Jane. By meeting separately, you are able to get more candid reporting. In addition, separate meetings initially are essential to identify and establish basic skills (such as active listening and validation) for each family member to help them use future sessions with their daughter productively.

In the early stages of the case (#2), it is better to start with a focus on psychoeducation about BPD and establishing yourself as both neutral and supportive to all (#3). The concept of a personality disorder is difficult and often confusing for parents to comprehend. Discussion and exploration of inherent temperament, genetic contribution, attachment issues, and parental "fit" open the door to a nonjudgmental, curious approach to thinking about their daughter. Parents are often hurt, shocked, and embarrassed by their borderline child's dramas, tantrums, and other out-of-control behaviors. Helping them to understand the basic concepts of emotion dysregulation and interpersonal hypersensitivity gives parents a foundation to help them develop a more skillful parental approach. Programs such as Family Connections, a free course offered through the National Education Alliance for Borderline Personality Disorder (NEABPD), and simple, clear information ("The BPD Brief"), and skills ("Family Guidelines") are extremely helpful and should be recommended at this point. All of these resources are available through the NEABPD website.

The timing around when and if you actually initiate family sessions (#4) is often driven by the emergence of a concrete issue usually involving finances or other practical matters. Many families have horror stories of family therapy gone terribly wrong, with much angry shouting and unresolved battles. The alliance and skill building you have done in advance separately with parents will help them handle the challenges of a family session more successfully and allow you to be more effective in refereeing the session.

Finally (#5), you can expect that Jane's problems have affected her brother. Just because he is "higher functioning" does not mean he does not have both confusion and emotion about the family dramas. Siblings are often suffering in silence as a way to put less burden on their parents. The resentment that comes from that strains the sibling relationship and furthers family tension. Encourage him to at least meet with you so you can get his perspective on the family dynamics and provide him some support and validation. Reminding the parents that he will understandably need their support is important.

Answers

1. U
2. U
3. H
4. H
5. U

Principles and Clinical Pearls

1. Learning about BPD will be the focal point of early sessions, during which you should help parents better understand how they can help their adult child with the disorder and avoid the pitfalls of judgment and criticism.
2. Often the BPD child's crises impact siblings in ways that are unexpressed; encouraging parents to remember to attend fully to all of their children is helpful and important.

Case Continues...

While Jane is attending twice-weekly therapy session with Dr. R and seeing a psychiatrist every 2 weeks to monitor the antidepressant she has started, the rest of the time she sleeps late, binge-watches online movies, eats junk food, and leaves her room and the house a mess. Her parents are alarmed at this development, to say the least. You proceed with a series of sessions with the parents designed to help them understand their daughter's behavior in light of what they are learning about BPD and working with them on developing more skillful ways of communicating and interacting with Jane. You refer to the Family Guidelines at every session.

You learn that Fred has a demanding job at a legal firm and is working long hours, in part to avoid dealing with Jane. Irene is a teacher who works close to home and often checks on Jane throughout the day. They are both moving from a frightened stance ("If we ask her to do more around the house, she says we are stressing her out. We don't want to worsen her depression!") to a more angry, externalizing position ("These meds are not working! We don't see her therapist helping her!")

While you encourage their open sharing of their fears and doubts, you also focus on concrete ways they can deal with Jane as their compassion is strained and their frustration grows.

Choice Point 3

You shift to a more practical approach and advise the parents that:

1. Jane needs them to become more demanding about household chores and keeping to a good daily schedule.
2. They provide more support and unconditional love, because Jane is struggling with more depression as she is coming to a deeper awareness of her situation.
3. They take a more balanced approach in responding, by noting that in many ways Jane is doing the best she can, AND they know she can do better - for example, by having more of a schedule.
4. You and they should have a conjoint session with Jane and her therapist to take a look at the progress Jane has made as well as the challenges that remain.
5. You schedule a family session to address parents' concerns with Jane.

Discussion

It is a very challenging point when parents are not seeing the progress they anticipated, and consequently question the efficacy of the treatment. Although you need to take their concerns seriously (sometimes there ARE problems in the therapy!), you also need to help them become better able to discuss their worries directly with Jane. Now is the time for parents to use their newly learned skills - can they listen to Jane's complaints without reacting, validate her concerns without dismissing or minimizing them, and resist joining her in blaming the therapy?

The notion that (#1) Irene and Fred can be effective if they just come down harder on Jane is wishful thinking. Young adults tend to regress at home, so bitterly fighting over household chores typically does not go well. This is indeed the time for Jane to build more structure, ideally with a real job. Household jobs simply do not have the built in accountability Jane needs to build self-confidence.

However, it is unwise for parents to continue to accept Jane's behavior for fear of stressing her out (#2). This must be seen as a vote of nonconfidence in Jane's ability to get back into a functional life. Their daughter will benefit from their belief that she can move forward, and parents need thoughtfully communicate this belief to influence Jane's course.

One productive way to address parental concerns about Jane's therapy is to have occasional conjoint sessions with Jane and her therapist (#4). With her therapist's support, Jane may be able to more fully speak to what she is working on in therapy and what is getting in the way of her moving forward. You and the therapist can also model how to discuss difficult impasses in treatment. In addition, it typically reassures parents to have contact with their family member's therapist, and improves understanding and confidence in the treatment. Encouraging the parents to use the session to ask how they can be most helpful/effective will help avoid the many pitfalls inherent in a conjoint session.

The conjoint session is also a way to prepare to move to a more classic family therapy (#5) yet at this point Fred, Irene, and Jane are all learning new skills that take time to master. Conjoint sessions can develop a shared confidence in the family's ability to have constructive conversations and manage emotion. This is preferable for having a first family session when frustration and hopelessness are high (#5). The family may not be ready to use the session well.

Answers

1. U
2. U
3. H
4. H
5. P

Principles and Clinical Pearls

1. Family therapy is a powerful tool best implemented when all have an awareness of the need to actively listen and observe, and manage their own reactivity. Validation is challenging to skillfully pull off when there is great conflict. Individuals with BPD, in their ambivalence about change and difficulty managing emotion, will lash out and deflect anticipated criticism by attacking and devaluing others. Parents are prime targets. Until parents are able to see their own contribution to their child's problems, family therapy will stall out.
2. The Family Guidelines highlight solid communication principles that simply and clearly illustrate how to best navigate a relationship with a family member with BPD. Developed by John Gunderson, M.D., and Cynthia Berkowitz, M.D., over 20 years ago, they continue to be extremely useful to families and should be thoroughly discussed in the initial stage of family involvement.

Case Continues...

With the support of Dr. R and encouragement from her parents, Jane gets a job in a small retail store. Irene is thrilled as she believes that fashion has always been a passion for Jane. However, there is not much foot traffic in the store, and Jane dislikes the manager who is "mean." Irene finds herself waking Jane up and nagging her to get to work on time. As it is summer, Irene is not teaching and puts her full effort into helping Jane, yet it appears that Jane is regressing in the face of her mother's increased availability.

Then, apparently overnight, Jane develops an intense, romantic relationship with a former high school friend, Art, who lives nearby with his parents. Art dropped out of community college and works at the local gas station. Jane looks brighter and less depressed, although she continues to struggle with her boss, often coming in late to work. When Jane is fired for unreliability, she blames it on her unreasonable boss. She subsequently spends all her time with Art, often staying overnight at his house.

Parents are extremely concerned. In addition to their anger over Jane's lack of responsibility toward her job, they also believe that Art is a bad influence. They suspect he smokes pot and has no ambition or future. Jane, however, is consumed by the relationship. Despite Irene's many efforts to engage her, Jane refuses to discuss what happened at the job and does not show any signs of looking for a new one.

After a honeymoon period, Jane and Art's relationship takes a darker turn. They are fighting more, and Jane confides in her mother numerous complaints about Art. No sooner does Irene carefully counsel Jane to end the relationship, they are back together. Parents are worried about the effects of the intense, unstable relationship on Jane's mood. They also find Jane's apparent obsession with Art disturbing. Parents' worst fears are realized when after yet another breakup, Jane takes a mild overdose of diphenhydramine. Jane admits to this after sleeping the day away. She calls her therapist and Irene drives her to a session that evening. She does not require medical care. Parents blame Art and want to forbid Jane to see him again.

Choice Point 4

You proceed to:

1. Inform Jane's parents that having intense, unstable relationships is part of having BPD and they need to accept it.
2. Recommend to your colleague that Jane needs to go into a higher level of care for her own safety.
3. Have a family session with Jane and her parents, in which you help Irene and Fred express (without blame or criticism) the effect the overdose had on them.
4. Have a team meeting with Dr. R, the psychopharmacologist, Jane, parents and yourself to discuss progress and problems.
5. Set up a series of family sessions to explore expectations of small steps forward that both Jane and parents jointly agree upon.

Discussion

While psychoeducation (#1) about BPD is invaluable in enhancing parents' understanding of the disorder, BPD should not be offered as an excuse for negative behaviors. However, parents do need to be realistic about what they can and cannot control. Unless Jane expresses suicidality and her therapist feels that she is at high risk, it is best that Jane continue working on her vulnerability in relationships in her outpatient therapy (#2). You can be a support to Dr. R as well in helping assess Jane's fluctuating level of risk over time.

The third choice highlights the way in which parents have an opportunity to help Jane to understand the effects of her impulsive actions on them. It is typical for parents to have post-traumatic stress symptoms around suicide attempts and high-risk behaviors. It is also a chance to be clear about how much they do care about Jane.

Having a team meeting (#4) may be helpful, yet also runs the risk of overly emphasizing the importance of the overdose. It may be better to see if Jane can regain ground and make positive moves forward.

This may be an important time to shift the focus from a problematic relationship, which Jane needs to work on in her individual therapy, to the overall situation at home (#5), Jane's parents cannot choose her boyfriends, however much they may want to. By focusing on Art as "the problem" they are more likely to inadvertently encourage the drama of the relationship by making it "forbidden." Instead, using collaboration to help Jane and parents find ways to share their concerns in a neutral, observing manner is preferable to parents making threats and ultimatums. The more effective stance for parents is to shift their focus away from Art and onto their need for Jane to have a more responsible daily structure.

Answers

1. U
2. U
3. H
4. P
5. H

Principles and Clinical Pearls

A marker of progress in therapy and parent skill development may be that patients and their families interact more as collaborators than constant adversaries.

Case Continues...

To the parents' consternation, Jane continues to see Art, explaining how he really wants "to be there" for her. More positively, she begins applying for a new job and takes a course at the local college. Jane willingly participates in the family session. Parents discuss their needs, such as knowing where Jane is every night by 9:00 (sometimes she stays at Art's) so they can get a good night's sleep. You alternate parent sessions with family sessions and coach Irene and Fred to continue to work more collaboratively with Jane. You emphasize that her expression of anger at them is progress, and that they should listen nondefensively and agree with any parts of her protestations that are valid. The parents are growing less critical and judgmental, and now avoid saying they want something "because it will be good for Jane." Jane responds positively to these developments.

However, you observe in the sessions a growing friction between Fred and Irene. You see Fred present in a condescending way toward Irene, often criticizing her for being "too easy and coddling" of Jane. Irene then gets defensive and points out that Fred's rigid sense of right and wrong has been the problem for Jane. Furthermore, Jane seems to exacerbate their differences by playing them against each other, particularly around money issues. You can see the tension between parents growing as it becomes clear that Jane decides that she is not ready to return to college in the fall, but rather will be staying home with them. Irene and Fred believe that this is best for Jane but start to argue more about logistics and finances.

Choice Point 5

Faced with this growing unrest, you:

1. Recommend that Fred and Irene see a couples therapist to work out their differences.
2. Help them examine their different parenting styles and consider the way Jane has often exploited those differences.
3. Minimize the marital tension by explaining that such conflict is normal when dealing with family problems.
4. Help Irene and Fred develop a clear financial plan for Jane to which they can both agree.
5. Recommend that limits being placed upon Jane should be explained and enforced by Irene, to help get Fred out of the critical role and into a more supportive role.

Discussion

Encountering marital friction while doing family work is unavoidable. Fred and Irene's fear and wish to control Jane will be activated by her classic borderline struggles with impulsivity, dichotomous thinking, and desperate longing for relationships. Because Jane needs to learn how to make good decisions for herself, parents need to manage their anxiety and resist striking out at her or each other.

Although ultimately the marriage may have deeper problems which require couples work (#1), referring them now misses the larger point of (#2) helping parents examine the differences in how they each see and respond to Jane's problems, and the wisdom in each view. Helping them achieve a wise middle path that combines support and limit setting is the more useful goal. Irene and Fred are then more likely to recognize the ways that Jane has maximized and distorted their different styles as a way to get what she desperately wants, and respond to her as a unified team.

This is another opportunity to observe the unique ways someone with BPD effects the entire family system in ways that are not "normal" (#3). Research from the Family Connections program shows that families who have a member with BPD experience greater "burden."

   This remains a valuable time to continue family work as Jane will likely continue to exploit her parents' relative weaknesses as she has done in the past. A potentially fruitful discussion may evolve if parents are coached to avoid defensiveness or minimization and be able to examine these patterns with their daughter. Identifying such dysfunctional patterns together can be the first step toward changing them. A concrete task (#4) like agreeing on financial plan (or a simple allowance amount) provides a tough but fruitful opportunity for Jane and parents to come together in a collaborative spirit. It is critical that Fred and Irene be consistent with the plan. As noted in Family Guideline #10, "Parental inconsistencies fuel severe family conflicts. Develop strategies that everyone can stick to." Anticipating how Jane may struggle with increased responsibility will help Irene and Fred to hold their position and see how their predictability helps Jane move forward.

   Finally, it appears that part of the conflict is fueled by a dynamic where Irene grows more supportive and protective toward Jane in reaction to Fred's criticism. Helping them shift roles by tasking Fred with increased validation and Irene with delivering the limits and "tough love" will help favorably shift these dynamics.

Answers

1. P
2. H
3. U
4. H
5. H

Principles and Clinical Pearls

1. In this stage of treatment, Jane is both making progress and still struggling to "catch up" to a functional life trajectory in sudden crisis, parents often pull together, but over the long haul, parents can vacillate from being hopeful and optimistic when things are good to being angry and pessimistic when they see their BPD loved one takes two steps back. This puts much strain on a marriage.
2. The very skills that parents are learning for their daughter's treatment should also be applied to their relationship with each other. Working together to hold a clear, compassionate, unified approach in the face of their daughter's challenges is a goal they can both embrace which may improve their marital relationship.

Case Continues...

Jane ends up breaking up with Art, and although this is deeply upsetting, she makes no suicide attempt. She has taken a part-time job at the nursing home where her grandmother resides. She describes really liking the job and feels very appreciated there. She successfully completed one course at the nearby college and is planning to take two next semester.

Although it is still challenging for Irene and Fred to resist trying to steer Jane into certain directions, they reserve their advice for the times Jane actually asks for it. The continued monthly family sessions provide a forum for problem solving and promoting increased connection between Jane and her parents. Important discussions take place, such as examining how Jane and her parents will know when she is ready to resume college full time. Setbacks are seen as opportunities to understand more deeply the ways in which Jane struggles. Irene and Fred are impressed by the difference in their relationship with Jane and each other that have occurred by embracing skills such as validation. Irene and Fred decide to become Family Connections trainers to pass on their experiences to other parents dealing with children with BPD.

Clinical Pearls

1. Having resources such as family connections and the family guidelines provides a focus on skills and understanding that hold both family and clinician in good stead. Progress is uneven in the treatment of BPD, and a strong knowledge base can help everyone hold steady in the face of drama and setbacks.
2. Families benefit from the support and feedback of other families that make the family connection program so effective and successful. Encourage parents and significant others to take the 12-week course, and ideally, they will eventually become trainers themselves and help proliferate this invaluable free service.

Summary of Clinical Approach

Families struggle with how to effectively support their BPD loved one. They may grow more critical or controlling – or, less frequently, inappropriately accommodating. Learning concrete skills like validation can help markedly with communication and make for a much more effective approach. Family therapy, per se, is rarely helpful until all the family members have the needed skills to react with curiosity and rueful recognition when hearing complaints from other members of the family. Instead, helping parents focus on being effective, understanding their loved one's experience, and remaining stable, predictable, and reliable in the face of crises can go a long way toward helping the family stabilize.

Family Guidelines

John Gunderson and Cynthia Berkowitz

Goals: Go Slowly
1. Remember that change is difficult to achieve and fraught with fears. Be cautious about suggesting that "great" progress has been made or giving "you can do it" reassurances. "Progress" evokes fears of abandonment.

2. Lower your expectations. Set realistic goals that are attainable. Solve big problems in small steps. Work on one thing at a time. "Big" goals or long-term goals lead to discouragement and failure.

Family Environment: Keep Things Cool
3. Keep things cool and calm. Appreciation is normal. Tone it down. Disagreement is normal. Tone it down, too.
4. Maintain family routines as much as possible. Stay in touch with family and friends. There is more to life than problems, so do not give up the good times.
5. Find time to talk. Chats about light or neutral matters are helpful. Schedule times for this as you need to.

Managing Crisis: Pay Attention But Stay Calm
6. Do not get defensive in the face of accusations and criticisms. However, unfair, say little and do not fight. Allow yourself to be hurt. Admit to whatever is true in the criticisms.
7. Self-destructive acts or threats require attention. Do not ignore. Do not panic. It is good to know. Do not keep secrets about this. Talk about it openly.
8. Listen. People need to have their negative feelings heard. Do not say "it isn't so." Do not try to make the feelings go away. Using words to express fear, loneliness, inadequacy, anger, or needs is good. It is better to use words than to act out on feelings.

Addressing Problems: Collaborate and Be Consistent
9. When solving a family member's problems, ALWAYS
   (a) involve the family member identifying what needs to be done
   (b) ask whether the person can "do" what is needed in the solution
   (c) ask whether they want you to help them "do" what is needed
10. Family members need to act in concert with one another. Parental inconsistencies fuel severe family conflicts. Develop strategies that everyone can stick to.
11. If you have concerns about medications or therapists' interventions, make sure that both your family member and his or her therapist/doctor know. If you have financial responsibility, you have the right to address your concerns to the therapist or doctor.

Limit Setting: Be Direct But Careful
12. Set limits by stating the limits or your tolerance. Let your expectations be known in clear, simple language. Everyone needs to know what is expected of them.

13. Do not protect family members from the natural consequences of their actions. Allow them to learn about reality. Bumping into a few walls is usually necessary.
14. Do not tolerate abusive treatment such as tantrums, threats, hitting, and spitting. Walk away and return to discuss the issue later.
15. Be cautious about using threats and ultimatums. They are a last resort. Do not use threats and ultimatums as a means of convincing others to change. Only give them when you can and will carry through. Let others – including professionals – help you decide when to give them.

Adapted from McFarlane W, Dunne E. Family psychoeducation and multi-family groups in the treatment of Schizophrenia. Directions in Psychiatry. 1991;11:20.

Maureen Smith received her graduate degree from Smith College School for Social Work and has worked for the past 29 years at McLean Hospital. Since 2000, she served as a Director of Family Services for The Adult Outpatient Personality Disorder Program and the Gunderson Outpatient Program. She retired from McLean in 2017 and is currently in Private Practice.

Borderline Personality Disorder with Narcissistic Features

13

Benjamin McCommon

Choice Point Index
1. Framing observations about narcissistic problems
2. Discussing self-esteem regulation with a patient
3. How narcissistic problems impact recommendations for work
4. Collaborating on decisions, even when pressured otherwise
5. Maintaining curiosity with self-esteem regulation problems

---

Case Introduction

Andrew is a 26-year-old man who has come to you because his girlfriend of 5 years insisted that he seeks treatment to address his lack of gainful employment, or else she eventually would break up with him. He tells you that he finished a master's program in education 3 years earlier and obtained a teaching position in a high school but was fired in the middle of the first semester after a heated argument with his school's principal over the best way to prepare his students for an upcoming state-mandated examination. When he felt criticized by his girlfriend for being fired, Andrew said that he sat on the window ledge of their upper story apartment. Terribly frightened, she called 911. He was discharged from the emergency room the next day to a day treatment program, where he spent the next 6 months even though he now calls it "completely useless." Since then, he has had a few interviews for teaching positions and has occasionally worked part time as a tutor. His girlfriend has been paying the rent; he receives intermittent financial support from his father.

B. McCommon, M.D.
Department of Psychiatry, Columbia University, New York, NY, USA
e-mail: bhm7@cumc.columbia.edu

© Springer International Publishing AG, part of Springer Nature 2018
B. Palmer, B. Unruh (eds.), *Borderline Personality Disorder*,
https://doi.org/10.1007/978-3-319-90743-7_13

Andrew describes chronic feelings of inferiority and depression with treatment that began in his teenage years when his parents were divorced. Although he continued to live in the same home in an affluent neighborhood with his mother and younger brother, financial circumstances were far more constrained, and he felt inadequate and envious of his friends and classmates. He calls his father "a narcissistic jerk" for being grudging about child support payments despite having significant wealth, and he says that he is determined to never be like him. During that period and over the next years, Andrew would bang his head against the wall repeatedly if he felt angry or low. Many times, he would cheat on girlfriends, including his current girlfriend, when he felt hurt by something that they said or did, and afterward, he would be plagued with shame.

He tells you about having tried many medications without any benefit. He speaks in a derogatory tone about past psychiatrists and therapists, emphasizing that none of them have helped, and he accuses them of applying rote techniques without really caring about him except for their income from treating him. Meeting most of the criteria, he had been diagnosed with borderline personality disorder (BPD) in addition to Major Depressive Disorder and been referred to a dialectical behavioral therapy (DBT) skills group. He is especially scornful telling you about that experience. Andrew agrees, however, that BPD is an accurate diagnosis for him. Abruptly, he becomes tearful and says that maybe *he* is the problem: that he is terrible and untreatable.

Choice Point 1

For each choice point, choose H: "helpful," U: "unhelpful or harmful," or P: "perhaps helpful, with reservations."

How would you make use of your understanding of the importance of narcissistic problems in Andrew's evaluation?

1. Avoid discussing it with him, because the lack of evidence-based treatments for narcissistic problems makes it not worth the risk of him becoming hurt or angry.
2. Avoid discussing it with him, because it would be preferable to develop more of a treatment alliance first.
3. Explain your concern that he may have narcissistic problems in addition to BPD, and suggest reviewing the DSM-5 criteria for narcissistic personality disorder (NPD) with him.
4. Introduce that you have noticed that he seems to have fluctuations in self-esteem with feelings of inferiority – low self-esteem being most prominent – and ask him what he thinks about this.

Discussion

Your initial evaluation is already full of valuable information. The presence of BPD may explain the lack of response to medications despite his history of major depressive disorder. In the evaluation, the patient has shown possible extremes of self-esteem at multiple points including: excessively low self-esteem characterized by shame, badness, inferiority, and envy; and excessively high self-esteem characterized by superiority, righteousness, and using others.

The comorbidity of BPD with other personality disorders is high, and although robust epidemiological data are lacking, NPD may be seen in 15% of BPD patients [1]. NPD is the most obvious type of narcissistic problem, characterized by grandiosity; it has been described as "thick-skinned" narcissism. The other major type of narcissistic problem is "thin-skinned" narcissism, characterized by vulnerability and fragility with somewhat more covert superiority and grandiosity [2]. This patient has the more vulnerable form of narcissism, perhaps at least partly explaining his nonresponse to DBT, an evidence-based treatment for BPD.

There is no current evidence-based treatment available for NPD or narcissistic problems. Expert opinion advises the adaptation of evidence-based treatments for BPD (considered to be a "near neighbor disorder") to address NPD and narcissistic problems [2]. Choice 1 is accurate about the lack of evidence-based treatments for narcissistic problems, but it is important to be aware of these problems to be able to address them with adapted treatments for BPD. As with BPD, it is best not to defer diagnostic efforts as described in Choice 2. Instead, a tactful inquiry about these problems may help a patient feel understood even in the initial meeting. Because terms such as "narcissism" and "narcissist" often have pejorative connotations, Choice 3 may be helpful for some patients as a form of collaboration in diagnosis but lead to a strong negative reaction in others. It is advisable to use language that most patients will find acceptable (such as "self-esteem fluctuations" in Choice 4) with a bid for feedback and participation from the patient [2].

Answers

1. U
2. U
3. P
4. H

Principles and Clinical Pearls

1. Narcissistic problems are common in BPD and can present in multiple ways, including with a prominence of inferiority and fragility notably different from NPD described in the DSM-5.
2. Evidence-based treatments for BPD can be adapted to address narcissistic issues.
3. Diagnostic discussion of narcissistic problems can be done using language that is more acceptable to the patient.

Case Continues…

Andrew readily agrees to the idea of self-esteem problems, especially inferiority and low self-esteem. When you tactfully ask him whether he thinks that there is any possible evidence of superiority or high self-esteem, even if hidden, he quickly refers to his girlfriend paying the rent and having cheated on her. Then, in a tone that is both somewhat plaintive and somewhat aggressive, he asks, "So, are you saying that I'm a narcissist just like my father?"

Choice Point 2

How would you respond to Andrew's pressing you on the question of whether you think he is a narcissist?

1. Reassure him that you do not, because you do not think he meets full DSM-5 criteria for NPD.
2. Confirm that even though you doubt he meets full DSM-5 criteria for NPD, you think he likely does have significant narcissistic problems.
3. Ask him what he means by "narcissist" preliminary to discussing with him how self-esteem problems can augment the interpersonal hypersensitivity of BPD.

Discussion

More important than obtaining agreement from a patient about the diagnosis of NPD or acceptance of the terms "narcissism" or "narcissist" is agreement about the presence of a self-esteem problem, and how it might be addressed in a potential treatment. Choice 1 may be accurate that the patient does not meet full criteria for NPD, but it would be incomplete to leave the patient's self-esteem problems unaddressed, especially given the past history of treatment failures to which the self-esteem problems likely contributed. Choice 2 acknowledges the presence of narcissistic problems, but many patients will experience the use of terms like "narcissistic" as attacking, leading to difficulty collaborating in a discussion of diagnosis and treatment. Choice 3 models effective collaboration with a patient, starting with curiosity and interest about their understanding of terms like "narcissist." This then naturally leads to the clinician being able to offer an understanding of self-esteem problems.

Clinicians without extensive training in specialty treatments for BPD can make use of the simplified approach to psycho-education about interpersonal hypersensitivity offered by good psychiatric management (GPM) for BPD [1], one of the evidence-based treatments for BPD. In the GPM model of interpersonal hypersensitivity, patients with BPD exist in a fragile state of "connectedness" that is constantly threatened by interpersonal stressors, especially feelings of being rejected by others. If a patient feels rejected, states of "feeling threatened" and "aloneness" can emerge, and unless the patient is rescued by support, "despair" may result, possibly requiring ER visits or hospitalization. Even when "connectedness" is restored by additional support or the containment of a hospital stay, this will always be a fragile state because it is based on an idealized view of others. In GPM for BPD, much of the work of psychotherapy is focused on helping patients to develop more effective interventions in this cycle of self-states.

This GPM model can be adapted for patients with narcissistic and self-esteem problems by discussing how they have *intra*personal hypersensitivity in addition to interpersonal hypersensitivity [3]. This can be explained as having excessively high internal standards that allow them to feel "connectedness" to themselves in an idealized way with elements of superiority. This is fragile, however, because any failure to meet these standards can lead to severe self-rejection. The movement from "connectedness" to "feeling threatened," "aloneness," or "despair," does not necessarily require the participation of someone else: it can happen entirely within the patient's mind. When "connectedness" to self is lost, feelings of inferiority and shame may flood the patient, and all standards, not just excessively high standards, may be abandoned. They may need the participation of another person (or the ER or hospital) to recover the fragile, idealized state of "connectedness." As in GPM for BPD, psychotherapy for narcissistic and self-esteem problems will focus on helping the patient find better solutions and coping strategies to interrupt this cycle of self-states.

Answers

1. U
2. P
3. H

Principles and Clinical Pearls

1. Diagnosis of narcissistic problems or NPD should be done collaboratively with the patient, and the patient's acceptance of the diagnosis may not be necessary if the patient accepts the importance of attention to self-esteem problems.
2. The model of interpersonal hypersensitivity to rejection in BPD can be modified for patients with significant self-esteem or narcissistic problems to include intrapersonal hypersensitivity to rejection, in which failure to meet internal high standards can lead to extreme self-rejection.

Case Continues...

Andrew agrees to a treatment that is focused on addressing interpersonal and intrapersonal hypersensitivities leading to problems in work and in his relationships. His girlfriend comes to his second session and seems concerned and supportive. At your next meeting, Andrew tells you that they had an argument. His supervisor at the study center where he has done part-time tutoring of community college students offered him a full-time clerical position. His girlfriend was angry that he plans to turn this job down because he feels a clerical role to be beneath his level of education. Afterward, he felt like banging his head, which he avoided, but he sent a text to a woman with whom he had been sexually involved 2 years earlier. He also mentions being contacted a month ago by a former colleague who is now in charge of substitute teachers for the local school district. She encouraged him to submit a resume directly to her. He has started to work on his resume many times but has made little headway on it. He wonders whether it would be best to work on communication skills with his girlfriend and put off the job search for now.

Choice Point 3

How would you respond to learning about Andrew's work opportunities?

1. Suggest he bring in a copy of his resume for you to look at together.
2. Let him know that it is okay to wait for a job opportunity that he finds to be acceptable, especially if he is having problems with girlfriend.
3. Tell him that his unwillingness to take a lower level job is probably a manifestation of his self-esteem problems and that it would be best for him to try to overcome his reluctance, especially because all work is worthwhile.
4. Bring up the possibility that although he is qualified for higher level jobs, it might be helpful for him to initially pursue a lower level job so that he can work on his interpersonal and self-esteem problems in a lower pressure setting.

Discussion

For patients who have narcissistic problems in addition to BPD, the importance of making efforts to address work problems may be even greater than for patients with BPD alone. Aside from a lack of functional improvement in work and relationships, they may also be less likely to have symptomatic improvement, possibly because successfully engaging in productive work is an important source of self-esteem for most people. It would be unwise to suggest waiting to address work problems as in Choice 2, especially because for most patients, it may be easier at first to tackle emotional problems in the work setting, which may not be as charged or stressful as problems in relationship settings. Although Choice 3 is accurate, it has a critical or moralizing tone that might turn some patients off, and it does not include an explanation of how the stimulus of work might help patients to address their underlying self-esteem problems. Choice 4 accurately describes a painful reality that patients with self-esteem problems often face: a lower level job (which itself can be a blow to self-esteem that will have to be managed in treatment) may be the best option initially.

The direct use of case management techniques including help and guidance in gaining employment (like jointly reviewing a resume as in Choice 1) is important for patients with BPD alone and for patients who also have narcissistic problems. A patient with self-esteem problems may avoid doing a resume because his work history does not meet his high internal standards. Similar to facing a lower level job in

Choice 4, the self-esteem blow of needing help on a resume may also have to be discussed in treatment.

Answers

1. H
2. U
3. P
4. H

Principles and Clinical Pearls

1. Patients with self-esteem problems are unlikely to improve in relationships prior to addressing their problems in work, and lower level work settings may be appropriate initially.
2. The use of case management techniques may be useful and even necessary for patients who seem to be capable of functioning at a higher level, and this can be conceptualized as self-esteem problems interfering with the expression of a patient's full talents and abilities.
3. Having self-esteem problems that lead to limitations can further worsen self-esteem and require attention in treatment.

Case Continues…

Andrew brings a draft of his resume to the next session. His sense of shame and humiliation at having a checkered work history seems to be alleviated by discussing these feelings with you. He quickly has ideas about how to complete a good enough resume. After the session, he sends the resume to his former colleague. He is invited for an interview and then is offered a position on the roster of substitute teachers. He is told that it likely could be a full-time equivalent job if he wants it to be. At a subsequent session, he is concerned about how demanding this teaching role might be, and he wonders if it might be better to pursue the clerical position at the study center, even though he feels it to be beneath him. Somewhat confrontationally, he asks you, "Which one should I take?"

Choice Point 4

How would you respond to Andrew's question about which job to take?

1. Advise him not to take a job below his level of education because that might exacerbate his feelings of inferiority and shame.

2. Advise him not to take the more demanding job because there might be a higher likelihood of failure that could exacerbate his feelings of inferiority and shame.
3. Suggest that it would better for you not to be the decision maker but for the two of you to review the pros and cons of each job opportunity.
4. Explain that you think he should make the choice because otherwise his sense of inferiority would be reinforced.

Discussion

Choice 1 avoids the difficult reality, as discussed previously, that lower level positions may make sense for patients to consider as initial work opportunities as they work on interpersonal and self-esteem problems that might make higher level positions more challenging. In addition, although supportive advice is often a component of successful treatments for BPD, clinicians must be careful not to assume a role of omniscience that patients may desperately want. They can elicit feelings of inferiority and shame that might lead us to respond in excessive ways ourselves. They may expect us to be perfectly knowledgeable and caring to help them meet impossible internal standards. It is important to address this as a problem because any help from you will only provide fragile support until you inevitably disappoint them with your lack of perfect knowledge and care. Choice 2 may contain an accurate assessment of risk, but along these lines, it would be best to help the patient decide whether he wants to take that risk or not. It is true, as described in Choice 4, that looking to others for decision making may provide only temporary relief and perpetuate ideas of weakness and inability that harm self-esteem in the longer run. However, Choice 4 does not offer the collaboration found in Choice 3 that helps patients not feel alone in their difficulties.

Answers

1. U
2. U
3. H
4. P

Principles and Clinical Pearls

1. Clinicians may struggle with feelings of inadequacy when confronted with the demands of patients with narcissistic and self-esteem problems.
2. Clinicians must be careful to avoid responses to patients that might reinforce expectations of perfect care.

Case Continues...

Andrew seems to be agreeable to the idea of working together to consider the pros and cons of each job opportunity. But he arrives at the next session looking hostile and withdrawn. When you ask about this, he angrily berates you for leaving him in the lurch with his job decision. He says the delay of a week might mean neither job is still available. He tells you he was so upset that he banged his head the night after your last session, and he sarcastically adds, "But don't worry, there's no injury, so you don't have to be concerned." He says that he cannot understand why he thought treatment with you would be any different, because now it seems as pointless as with everyone else before.

Choice Point 5

How would you respond to Andrew's outburst?

1. Discuss with him how he is being overly hopeless and aggressive, and seems to be forgetting how he has benefited from working collaboratively with you in the past.
2. Apologize for not answering his question, and now tell him what you think would be the best job for him to take.
3. Apologize for not answering his question, but reiterate that you do not think giving a direct answer is in his best interest.
4. Express concern about his anger toward you, and wonder whether his anger may be an understandable consequence of feeling unrescued by you from a difficult decision.
5. Acknowledge his anger, and ask him to tell you more about how you disappointed him before inquiring about any changes in his self-esteem associated with his anger.

Discussion

The model of interpersonal hypersensitivity in BPD predicts that patients will have strong negative reactions when their state of fragile "connectedness" is lost. These include anger, devaluation, and help-rejection. Although Choice 1 is accurate, by itself it may not provide enough concern and support to be heard by a hostile, withdrawn patient. Clinicians should be comfortable apologizing to patients as demonstrated in Choices 2 and 3. This is especially important in working with patients who have significant self-esteem problems because it reminds them that you are not perfect, in addition to modeling for them comfortable acknowledgement of one's imperfections. However, Choice 2 represents an abandonment of collaborative decision making in the face of the patient's anger. When a patient expresses contempt, rage, and domination toward us, we may react with feelings of shame, inferiority, and submission. Ideally, we will try to be aware of these feelings, as well as any covert contempt, rage, and domination which these patients are likely also to elicit in us. Awareness and acceptance of these challenging feelings in ourselves help us to avoid acting in overly submissive or dismissive ways. Choice 2 probably includes an attitude of submission in reaction to the patient's anger, and Choice 1 may contain a small amount of reactive dismissiveness. Choice 3 accurately repeats your concern about decision making, but Choice 4 is best because it expresses concern as well as empathically and nonjudgmentally inviting an exploration of why the patient might have become angry with you.

Choice 4 allows revisiting the model of interpersonal and intrapersonal hypersensitivity with the patient. Patients who are angry may still be able to listen, although perhaps grudgingly. An example of a more complete response, during which you would be attentive to the patient's verbal and nonverbal reactions, might be:

"You hold yourself to very high standards, and so this choice can be very difficult. On the one hand, you are drawn to the higher level job because you expect to feel bad otherwise. On the other hand, you are afraid it will be too challenging for you. And the reality is that there is no way to know what is the perfect decision, and I'm guessing that this is leaving you indecisive. I think you're probably hoping I can save you from this difficult problem, but I can only help you make your decision as best as possible. And I think this leaves you really disappointed with me. You don't just hold yourself to high standards, you can hold other people to them, too, including me. And that means that when we are disappointing to you, you can feel that we are useless as you can feel yourself to be useless. I think this is a problem for us to work on, because when there is something that is not perfect but maybe just okay, you can completely dismiss it as no good at all. What do you think?"

Choice 5 is also appropriate and may lead to the same points made in the paragraph above; but it demonstrates slightly more curiosity about the self-esteem fluctuations underlying the anger. Further questions emerge from the assumption that making a choice between two equally viable (but imperfect) options led to an important internal experience that elicited rage and avoidance. The session could focus on that experience, including what Andrew imagines are your motives in having suggested a pro/con approach to examine his problems . For example, if Andrew imagines that you are critical of him for his indecision and is reacting defensively, you may want to make your position more clear. You might reassure him that acknowledging a problem can feel like a criticism, but your goal is to help. Or if Andrew imagines that you stop caring about him when he struggles with indecision, you could look at how his perception of you fluctuates along with his self-esteem. Helping him to learn how to recognize these fluctuations – and his changing experience of other people in these moments – could be quite helpful.

Answers

1. P
2. U
3. P
4. H
5. H

Principles and Clinical Pearls

1. Clinicians are likely to experience feelings similar to those in their patients, including both devalued and inflated states. It is important for the clinician to be aware (and accepting) of these feelings to minimize acting out on them and to have a chance to use them in helping patients understand their own difficulties.
2. The model of interpersonal (and intrapersonal) hypersensitivity is useful in examining difficult treatment interactions with patients who have narcissistic and self-esteem problems.

Summary of Clinical Approach

This case illustrates important principles of treating patients with BPD and narcissistic problems. Initial assessments should include evaluation and discussion of narcissistic and self-esteem problems, using language that is acceptable to patients. This allows treatment planning that considers evidence-based treatments for BPD, adapted for focusing on difficulties related to narcissism and self-esteem fluctuations. For clinicians without specialty BPD training, the most useful treatment approach may be built on the model of interpersonal hypersensitivity in BPD. This simplified approach can be modified to address intrapersonal hypersensitivity, in which patients reject themselves (and others) when they fail to meet excessively high internal standards. This treatment builds on principles helpful for patients with BPD alone, including use of case management techniques, emphasis on collaboration, focus on work functioning initially, and examination of problems using the lens of interpersonal hypersensitivity. The concept of intrapersonal hypersensitivity provides guidance in difficult treatment situations that arise when patients elicit powerful reactions in their treating clinicians.

References

1. Gunderson JG, Links P. Handbook of good psychiatric management for borderline personality disorder. Washington, DC: American Psychiatric Publishing; 2014.
2. Caligor E, Levy KN, Yeomans FE. Narcissistic personality disorder: diagnostic and clinical challenges. Am J Psychiatry. 2015;172(5):415–22.

3. Bernanke J, McCommon B. Training in good psychiatric management for borderline personality disorder in residency: an aide to learning supportive psychotherapy for challenging-to-treat patients. Psychodyn Psychiatry. 2018;46(2):181–200

Dr. McCommon is an assistant clinical professor of psychiatry at Columbia University. He is a teacher of Good Psychiatric Management for borderline personality disorder at Columbia University and of transference focused psychotherapy at Columbia University and New York University. He is a therapist in an ongoing study of extended treatment with transference-focused psychotherapy at the Personality Studies Institute and Weill Cornell Medical Center in New York. He was the director of a clinic for LGBT patients in the department of psychiatry at Columbia University and has written about sexual orientation issues and personality disorders.

Narcissistic Personality Disorder with Borderline Features

14

Elsa Ronningstam

Choice Point Index
1. Responding to patients' early doubts about therapist competence and threatening/controlling behavior
2. Inquiring about the patients' reasoning and understanding of why they seek treatment and what they expect and want from treatment
3. Discussing the NPD diagnosis and the optimal way of initiating and timing this
4. Attention to and exploration of the patient's emotional functioning and capability
5. Attention to external life experiences (occurring outside of treatment) that can contribute to corrective emotional experiences and realizations, which support and encourage change

---

Case Introduction

Carol is a 28 year-old married woman and a second-year student in law school, with a plan to become a lawyer like her husband, father, and grandfather. She was referred to you for psychotherapy after discharge from a psychiatric hospital where she was admitted after a serious, near-lethal suicide attempt, the first in her life. She was also referred to couple's therapy and part of your treatment contract was to establish ongoing collaborative communication between you and the couple's therapist. Her husband, 9 years her senior, is the owner and president of a law firm specialized in corporate law. As your therapy sessions begin, she is back home living with him and has resumed her full-time studies in law school.

14

E. Ronningstam, Ph.D.
Harvard Medical School, Department of Psychiatry, McLean Hospital, Belmont, MA, USA
e-mail: ronningstam@email.com

© Springer International Publishing AG, part of Springer Nature 2018
B. Palmer, B. Unruh (eds.), *Borderline Personality Disorder*,
https://doi.org/10.1007/978-3-319-90743-7_14

163

At the first session, Carol tells you that over the past 10 years she has been in intermittent psychotherapy with three different therapists, but does not believe in therapy because her previous therapists were naïve and dismissive, and she felt blamed and unsupported. Nevertheless, she agreed to see you for a while, primarily to please her husband and because committing to psychotherapy had been a condition for her discharge from the hospital. She felt challenged by the fact that she survived her effort to end her life, especially since she had thoroughly prepared her suicide. She expressed difficulties with accepting that she now has to face her life and its problems, which had been overwhelming and embarrassing to her. Halfway into the session, Carol looks at you with critical, resentful, distant eyes and says: "So you think you can help me ... the other therapists thought so, too, but I came to realize they just made it worse for me. I have extensive legal knowledge, and if you screw up with me, I will sue you!"

Choice Point 1

For each intervention, choose H: "helpful," U: "unhelpful or harmful," or P: "perhaps helpful, with reservations."

How do you respond to Carol's statement of threat and challenge?

1. Close the case and ask her to leave.
2. Inform her that you have your own lawyer for your legal protection and that none of your previous patients have ever pursued a lawsuit against you.
3. Tell her that psychotherapy can be a tough and challenging process and that her negative experiences in the past obviously have affected her, made her cautious, and mobilized her needs to protect and defend herself.
4. Request that her husband join the next session and establish a contractual agreement that precludes lawsuits.
5. Inquire about her experiences with previous therapists, and invite her to describe what went wrong and her own understanding as to how and why.
6. Make a patient-centered interpretation pointing out that she is afraid of starting psychotherapy and addressing the difficulties leading to her suicide attempt. Suggest that she perceives you as a negative threat and needs to keep her distance and control, avoid discussing her own feelings and problems, which could risk her feeling overpowered by you, and as a means of self-protection she is threatening to sue you.

Discussion

Starting psychotherapy can be a very challenging experience for patients with pathological narcissism (PN) or NPD that readily evokes negative anticipations of competition, subordination, being overpowered, and losing control. These experiences trigger defensive self-enhancing and aggressive interpersonal reactions and sometimes extreme efforts to take charge of the therapeutic process. Assuming the therapists' malevolence or incompetence can represent a dismissive and avoidant attachment pattern that is common in NPD, an overreaction to the therapist's facial expressions, or a projection of patients' own anger, shame, or incompetence.

If you take these patients' initial threatening or controlling interactions at face value and respond by trying to elicit more socially appropriate behavior, you may inadvertently evoke shame or a self-enhancing conviction that you are out to confine or defeat them. You also risk falling into the trap of getting entrenched into their efforts to create a sensation-seeking, self-enhancing initial drama that can effectively steer your attention away from their actual problems. NPD patients tend to use interpersonal provocations to redirect attention from the actual purpose of the session and treatment in general.

This initial phase can be critical for alliance-building. It is important that therapists position themselves in a way that both acknowledges the patients' prior and current reactions (specifically those related to narcissistic pathology and self-regulation), but also points to the purpose of treatment and the specific role of the therapist [11]. Taking patients' threats concretely (choices 1, 2, and 4) runs counter to alliance-building and may only escalate aggression, distrust, and risk for dropout.

Patients with PN or NPD often present themselves in ways that differ from their internal subjective feelings and experiences. They tend to neglect social and interpersonal rules and be less aware of undesirable or provocative aspects of their behavior. This scenario easily invites therapists to engage in enactments by making assumptions about the patients' intentions, or by interpreting or labeling their behavior as pathological. This may confirm the patients' negative expectations of treatment and escalate their efforts to self-enhance or maintain control by distancing themselves and dismissing the therapist. Consequently, it is essential that the therapists pay attention to and manage their own reactions and countertransference while at the same time attending to their patients' expressions of pathological narcissism and related experiences in order to tactfully manage these initial challenges in this early process of building the alliance.

Interpretations (choice 6) are generally not useful at an early stage when patients are entrenched in and preoccupied with their own projections, explanations, and anticipations. They can even cause harm by escalating patients' negativity toward the therapist and reinforcing aggressive relational barriers. Interpretations are best delivered when a therapeutic alliance has been established [2] and the patient shows some spontaneous curiosity about the nature of the interaction with the therapist and has achieved some distance from its immediacy [3]. Early interventions should focus on providing psychoeducation, reality-anchored brief explanations, and validation in order to help the patient gain a more adaptive sense of control over their own emotional difficulties within the treatment. Ongoing explorations of their reasoning and experiences at a deeper level over time can help them develop a sense of self-agency and reflective ability.

Answers

1. U
2. U
3. H
4. U
5. P
6. U

Principles and Clinical Pearls

1. Managing patients' initial provocations and challenging the treatment by respect-
   fully and non-judgmentally inquiring about their reasoning and understanding of
   why they seek treatment and what they expect and want from treatment, and
   clarifying the purpose and process of treatment.

   Attend to the difference between patients' external presentation and their
   internal subjective experiences and struggle.

Case Continues...

You encourage Carol to describe her concerns about starting a new therapy, especially given her past negative experiences in treatment. In response to this intervention, she takes a deep breath and remains silent for a moment before looking up at
you and saying: "Yes, I appreciate that you can see that ... none of my previous
therapists could help me understand myself, and that has made me feel increasingly
lonely and very hopeless, though I don't understand why." You ask her what was
missing, and she spends the next sessions describing more in detail her experience
of her previous treatment – how she felt past therapists criticized or ignored her
problems and especially her needs and efforts to secure her self-esteem and control
by eliminating fluctuating and unpredictable aspects of her functioning. She also
describes the events and experiences leading up to her suicide attempt, including
failing an exam for the first time in her life and her subsequent profound shame. She
expresses a deep distrust of others as well as a sense that they lack understanding
and caring intentions toward her.

As the treatment is unfolding, you notice that Carol is very preoccupied with and
enclosed within herself, as if there is no one else there listening and responding to
her. You also notice her tendencies to dismiss whoever might be there for her,
including yourself. You feel like Carol does not consider that her words are having
any effect upon you.

Choice Point 2

How would you respond to Carol's self-encapsulation and active efforts to distance herself from others, including you?

1. Point out that she seems to reject everybody around her, including you, and that this tendency must have made her overlook previous therapists' efforts to help her.
2. Point out how her experiences of feeling dismissed and misunderstood cause her to be distrustful of others, which in turn may increase her sense of being in control, and while this can temporarily help her feel strong and independent, it has also a negative long-term impact as it keeps her disconnected from others and alone.
3. Explore further her understanding of how and why this pattern of distrusting others and feeling dismissed by them has unfolded in her life, and how currently it affects her.
4. Tell her that you feel so sorry to hear about her difficult experiences with previous therapists, and that you will do your best to try to understand and help her.
5. Inform her that if she is not capable of or interested in trusting and collaborating with you, she will not be able to change her life and she will continue to be at risk for suicide.

Discussion

Altering and balancing between validating patients' accounts of their experience and continuing exploration of their perspectives and experiences is important for deepening the alliance and building the patients' confidence, trust, and capacity to relate to the therapist.

As alliance-building continues, it is important to engage patients' sense of agency and self-reflective ability in deepening a shared understanding of patterns in their self-regulatory and interpersonal functioning (choices 2 and 3). It is also important to focus on their fluctuating self-esteem. This stance can gradually bring about a nonjudgmental recognition of patients' self-enhancing, superiority-asserting, and controlling interpersonal patterns as well as their underlying avoidance, fear, and insecurity. For example, therapists may comment that a specific experience sounds "challenging," "difficult," or "unexpected" to convey an understanding of its effect on the patient. This can encourage the patients' sense of ownership of their experiences, which also promote their sense of agency and ability to reflect and process within the therapeutic alliance. In addition, such strategy can also prevent the therapists to "merge" or "over-empathize" with the patient, which can increase the risk for evoking patients' overwhelming intolerable emotions and reflective collapse.

However, therapists can also at this point become impatient at feeling dismissed and experience retaliatory frustration and urges to criticize the patient by pointing out that they do not seem to make any efforts to relate and engage, but just complain and blame others while prioritizing their own perspectives (choices 1 and 5). On the other hand, therapists can also express too much empathy or sympathy with patients' grievances (choice 4). Neither of these approaches is useful at this point, as each of them in different ways would steer attention away from patients' core problems with self-esteem, identity, suicidality, and attachment.

Answers

1. U
2. P
3. H
4. U
5. U

Principles and Clinical Pearls

1. Using relatively "neutral" validating language can help patients feel that their difficulties are being recognized at a basic level while the therapist is also inviting deeper reflection and understanding of their subjective experiences.

Case Continues...

Carol suddenly raises the question of whether you think she has a NPD, and she seems very defensive and aggressive in describing how her previous therapists had "thrown that into [her] face." This made her feel very hopeless, especially as she came across certain media declaring it an untreatable condition. She also mentions the couple's therapist has recently tried to convince her husband that her NPD was the cause of all the problems between them. Carol points out, however, that in the hospital she had been diagnosed with major depressive disorder and possible bipolar disorder, which she found less humiliating although it pointed toward a very gloomy future. She looks at you aggressively straight in the eyes and asks what you think.

Choice Point 3

How do you respond when Carol demands your opinion about whether she has NPD?

1. You feel provoked, and tell her she obviously has NPD in addition to some borderline traits, and that she has to come to terms with this being a lifelong condi-

tion with very little chance of changing, especially if she continues treatment the way she is now.

2. You feel concerned and afraid of Carol's potential threatening impulsivity and aggression, and say that she does not have NPD at all and that all the other therapists assigning her this diagnosis are wrong and inappropriate.
3. Suggest that you and Carol take this opportunity to discuss the diagnostic issue in its full complexity by reviewing both the trait and dimensional criteria for NPD in DSM-V (Section II and III), clearing up common misconceptions and misunderstandings about the diagnosis, highlighting the discrepancy between internal experiences and external interpersonal presentations, and individually tailoring appropriate aspects of the diagnosis to Carol's specific experience of her difficulties.
4. Tell Carol you do not find the NPD diagnosis useful and suggest she go online and research it for herself, then come back with any questions she may have.

Discussion

The NPD diagnosis has a particularly negative connotation among psychiatric disorders, even when compared with other personality disorders. Both the media and the psychiatric and psychotherapeutic community contribute to this pall over NPD. Patients readily perceive the NPD diagnosis as an unfair, devaluing, or critical accusation, or as a paradoxically self-enhancing property ("I have NPD so you will not be able to treat me"). Consequently, giving the diagnosis without proper explanations, clarifications, and adjustments tends to backfire and evoke strong negative reactions (choice 1). Avoiding any evaluation or discussion of this diagnosis (choices 2 and 4) can also have a negative effect on the therapeutic process.

Despite these potential pitfalls, therapists working with NPD patients have a unique opportunity to explain, clarify, and demystify the diagnosis as a potentially informative descriptor of patients' struggles (choice 3). By integrating the proposed dimensional model for NPD in Section III of DSM-5 with the established nine trait criteria in Section II, the diagnostic criteria and descriptions of the dimensions related to identity, self-direction, empathy, and intimacy can then be discussed and adjusted to the patient's own understanding of their problems [1]. Also helpful is to clarify how NPD can co-occur with other disorders, such as depression, bipolar disorder, and (in Carol's case) the traits of impulsivity, and affective and interpersonal instability in BPD.

Answers

1. U
2. U
3. H
4. U

Principles and Clinical Pearls

1. Discussion about the NPD diagnosis is best deferred until patients are ready for, and/or themselves initiate a discussion about the diagnosis with a request for the therapist's opinion. The interaction should be carried out in an informative and systematic manner seeking to link what is known about NPD and its treatment with patients' own understanding of their difficulties, as it otherwise can turn aggressive, dismissive, or blaming.

Case Continues...

The treatment deepens after a careful discussion of the NPD diagnosis that helps Carol feel as though her core difficulties are more understood by both her and you. Carol becomes more collaborative in the treatment and reflects more deeply on how her decision to become a lawyer relates to her family background and to feeling alone. She is the oldest of three sisters and her mother was a housewife. As the first daughter in the family, Carol was met with high parental expectations and appreciation of her intelligence, eloquence, and decisiveness. From early on, she felt it was assumed that she would join her father as a partner in his law firm. As an emerging adult in college, she began to struggle more intensely with self-esteem and had bouts of acute insecurity alternating with impressive achievements such as running marathons, biking across the country, and rock-climbing. She felt increasingly unhappy and alone until she met the man she married, and for a while she felt more accomplished just by virtue of becoming his wife. She also decided to pursue law school, which she had postponed doing for several years. As you are listening carefully to this story you get a very heavy, unpleasant sense in your chest and stomach, and wonder what this could represent.

You get a call from the couple's therapist who reports Carol just informed her husband that she has been intimately involved with another man over the past few weeks. This is her first episode of infidelity and it prompted her adoring husband, who feels he devoted his life to supporting her, to become extremely upset, feel betrayed, and threaten a divorce. The couple's therapist insists that Carol should be confronted about her hurtful behavior, take responsibility, and request her husband's forgiveness. Carol has not told you anything about this affair.

Choice Point 4

How should you address having learned about Carol's infidelity directly with her?

1. Inform her that you got a phone call from the couple's therapist mentioning her recent extramarital affair and suggest a joint session with her husband and the couple's therapist.

2. Confront her for withholding such important information and for not using the psychotherapy to process her role and experiences of her marriage, and point out her aggression and avoidance of her emotions in hiding this material from you.
3. Ask whether and how her recent reflection on her background and complex experiences of her identity, self-esteem, and future may have affected her in some way that motivated this sudden engagement in an affair.
4. Inquire about her own understanding of why she has engaged in an affair now, in the context of her recent focus during sessions on issues of identity and managing expectations as a lawyer and in her marriage.

Discussion

Patients with NPD can be quite detached from their own feelings and often not aware of the feelings they evoke in others. They can present with an eloquent verbal plasticity and ability to describe and express emotions but still remain disconnected in a more substantive way from their own and others' emotions and reactions. This disconnect can be caused either by a more or less conscious motivation to avoid, preserve control, or enhance oneself by redirecting attention away from emotions, or by an inability to recognize, feel, or tolerate one's own and others' feelings. Clinical and empirical studies of NPD have identified deficits in emotion processing, including low emotion tolerance and alexithymia (impairment in identifying and describing feelings in words, or in differentiating feelings from bodily sensations caused by emotional arousal). Overly rigid self-orientation, narcissistic defensiveness, and lack of imagination and symbolization can also contribute to these difficulties [5, 6]. In addition, unprocessed emotional narcissistic trauma can cause an inability to access certain emotions, which can be somatized or psychophysiologically contained in the body [4, 8, 10]. As a consequence, interactions between NPD patients and therapists can become disengaged from any matching, attuned, or appropriate emotional expressions related to what is being discussed.

In these situations, therapists can become engulfed by their own experiences and reactions that in some way correspond to patients' verbally articulated but emotionally detached accounts [9]. Psychophysiological reactions in therapists, for example, may provide hints about patients' non-explicit, non-verbalized internal struggles.

When internal struggles are not sufficiently verbalized in individual therapy, it is important to assess whether there is a need for additional structure and accountability, such as by recommending adjunctive family, couples, or group therapy. This is especially true with regard to patients like Carol with comorbid borderline traits of impulsivity and interpersonal symptom enactment, and patients who may otherwise keep hidden comorbid substance use, eating disorders, or other self-destructive behaviors. Adjunctive avenues of accountability and confrontation may be conjoined to or referenced within the individual therapy (choice #1 and #2). Introducing these additional structures is more strongly indicated if you perceive a high risk in allowing unverbalized conflicts and associated unreported behavior to persist without active monitoring and confrontation. However, imposing these requirements too early and in the absence of a strong alliance may be too provocative and overwhelming, causing patients to escalate narcissistic self-enhancement through defensive aggression or dismissiveness.

Most essential within the context of individual therapy is to give NPD patients space and encouragement to begin to sort out and verbalize previously unmetabolized struggles (choice #4). It may be helpful to relate interpersonal and behavioral enactments (e.g., Carol's affair) to current developments within the therapy, if this is done tentatively so as not to outpace patients' own capacities for reflection (choice #3).

Answers

1. U
2. U
3. P
4. H

Principles and Clinical Pearls

1. Pay specific attention to and explore the patient's emotional functioning and capability. Do not automatically assume that emotional disengagement represents a self-enhancing defense strategy or deliberate unwillingness to engage and relate. It may instead reflect genuine alexithymic or other neuropsychological deficits in emotional processing, or relate to compartmentalized emotional narcissistic trauma.

Case Continues...

In response to your inquiry about the affair, Carol starts to cry and for the first time you sense she is emotionally genuinely engaged in the alliance and able to address her deep sense of insecurity and confusion regarding who she is and what she wants for herself. She describes having held on to the idea of becoming a lawyer to please her father and get his support. At the same time, as a young girl she already felt engulfed and threatened by her mother's way of functioning. She came from a lower socioeconomic background and found it specifically difficult to adjust to a new and more upscale social and cultural environment. In addition, she also struggled with intense fluctuations in temper and mood.

Carol had always felt alone and torn by a need to support her father and control and minimize the embarrassments she associated with her mother. She felt oppressed by her mother's neediness and unable to help her. Meeting her husband-to-be had initially seemed a confirmation of her worth and provided relief, but as the marriage progressed and she sensed her husband's aspirations for her to pursue law school and have children, Carol had felt increasingly overwhelmed, confused, unhappy, worthless, and – for the first time in her life – suicidal. When she failed an exam in law school, the decision to end her life seemed unavoidable as such a letdown had never happened before. Within weeks and without revealing her experience to anybody, she researched and decided on a plan that according to her evaluation would have a minimal risk to fail. She now tells you that since discharge from the hospital, she has continued to consider this plan despite its initial failure. However, she has also noticed that her extramarital affair has somewhat lessened her suicidal preoccupations and helped her feel more hopeful about her future. She also feels guilty for cheating on her husband, whom she still appreciates for his love and support.

Choice Point 5

Where do you focus the treatment, given these new developments?

1. Acutely manage this disclosure of ongoing suicidal ideation by requiring Carol to return to the hospital or sign up for an intensive outpatient program in order to continue treatment with you.
2. Validate the confusing nature of her gradual changes and the escalating discomfort in her marriage, and explore her understanding of each.
3. Explore her understanding of the shifts in her suicidality in response to failing her exam and engaging in the affair, and how it all might relate to her husband's suggestion that she pursue law school and have children.
4. Tell her that her affair is symptomatic of her NPD-related tendency to impulsively enact her problems interpersonally, and suggest she work on learning skills to control such impulses.
5. Focus on the exploration of her difficulties with female identity development and her complex relationships with both her mother and father.

Discussion

The fact that Carol has reached a point where she is able to feel sad, cry, and address her insecurity and confusion with you represents a major step forward in treating her NPD, and a good prognostic sign. Further exploration of Carol's decision to pursue a relationship with a new man can lead to further self-reflection and insights about the nature of her difficulties and clarification of her own future goals. It is crucial to differentiate between whether her affair represents primarily an impulsive symptom enactment, arising out of self-enhancement and avoidance, or whether it indeed may be a corrective relational and emotional experience of a different type than her marriage, which potentially can help to consolidate some sense of identity and capacity for intimacy [7]. It is useful to evaluate her suicidal ideation over time to help her differentiate genuine intent to die from normative experiences of sadness, grief, loss, and feeling overwhelmed from the changes that are underway.

Answers

1. U
2. P
3. H
4. U
5. P

Principles and Clinical Pearls

1. Experiences of being seen, validated, or understood represent important progress in psychotherapy with patients with NPD and can evoke normative sadness and grief as well as escalate suicidal ideation, requiring careful and non-reactive evaluation.
2. External life experiences (occurring outside of treatment) can contribute to corrective emotional experiences and realizations that can support and encourage change.

Case Concludes...

After one and a half years of psychotherapy, Carol decided to postpone a decision about a career as a lawyer. Instead, she got a full-time job teaching rock climbing to middle- and high-school students, which she finds deeply gratifying. She divorced her husband and pursued a relationship with the man she met while still married. She feels still intermittently confused and bothered by her difficulties consolidating a sense of identity and future plans. She also struggles with self-esteem fluctuations and difficulties tolerating and understanding her emotions, but she no longer felt suicidal or preoccupied with suicidal plans. She feels more hopeful and able to engage in relationships and interactions with others, especially her new intimate relationship.

Summary of Clinical Approach

Patients with a primary NPD with accompanying borderline features present with specific challenges in psychotherapy. Their initial provocations and dismissiveness can significantly mask their internal struggle. A neutral therapeutic approach with intermittant validation of subjective experiences can help patients feel seen and recognized, invite accounts of their own perspectives and engage their reflective ability.

Exploration of emotional functioning and capability is important as emotional disengagement can represent both a self-enhancing defense strategy or a neuropsychological deficit in emotional processing. Attention to external life experiences outside of treatment is also important as they can contribute to corrective emotional experiences and realizations promoting change.

References

1. American Psychiatric Association. Diagnostic and statistical manual of mental disorders. 5th ed. Arlington: American Psychiatric Association; 2013.
2. Gabbard GO, Horwitz L, Allen JG, Frieswyk S, et al. Transference interpretation in the psychotherapy of borderline patients: a high-risk, high-gain phenomenon. Harv Rev Psychiatry. 1994;2(2):59–69.
3. Kernberg OF, Selzer MA, Koenigsberg HW, Carr AC, Appelabum AH. Psychodynamic psychotherapy of borderline patients. New York: Basic Books, Inc. Publishers; 1989. p. 104–5.
4. Maldonado JL. Vicissitudes in adult life resulting from traumatic experiences in adolescence. Int J Psychoanal. 2006;87(5):1239–57.
5. Ronningstam E. Pathological narcissism and narcissistic personality disorder – recent research and clinical implications. Curr Behav Neurosci Rep. 2016;3(1):34–42. https://doi.org/10.1007/s40473-016-0060-y.
6. Ronningstam E. Intersect between self-esteem and emotion regulation in narcissistic personality disorder – implications for alliance building and treatment. Borderline Personality Disorder and Emotion Dysregulation. 2017;4(3):1–13. https://doi.org/10.1186/s40479-017-0054-8.
7. Ronningstam E, Gunderson J, Lyons M. Changes in pathological narcissism. Am J Psychiatry. 1995;152:253–7.
8. Simon RI. Distinguishing trauma-associated narcissistic symptoms from posttraumatic stress disorder: a diagnostic challenge. Harv Rev Psychiatry. 2001;10:28–36.
9. Tanzilli A, Muzi L, Ronningstam E, Lingiardi V. Countertransference when working with narcissistic personality disorder: an empirical investigation. Psychotherapy. 2017;54(2):184–94.
10. Van der Kolk B. The body keeps the score. Brain, mind and body in the healing of trauma. New York: Penguin Book; 2014.
11. Weinberg I, Ronningstam E. Examination of factors contributing to improvement in NPD patients in psychotherapy. 14th Congress of the International Society for Study of personality disorders; Montreal, Canada, October, 2015.

Dr. Ronningstam is an Associate Professor at Harvard Medical School, Department of Psychiatry, and a Clinical Psychologist at McLean Hospital, affiliated with the Gunderson Outpatient Program. She is also a member of the American Psychoanalytic Association and on the faculty of the Boston Psychoanalytic Society and Institute. Her primary specialty is diagnosis and treatment of narcissistic personality disorder (NPD). Over the past 30 years, she has authored over 90 publications, including several textbooks and educational guidelines on NPD, and has given over 150 presentations, lectures, and courses both nationally and internationally. As a member of the Boston Suicide Study Group and the Advisory Board of the American Foundation for Suicide Prevention Boston Chapter, Dr. Ronningstam is active in initiatives focused on identifying, treating, and preventing suicide.

Providing Consultation to Organize Specialist Treatment

15

Joan Wheelis

Choice Point Index
1. Initiating consultation for a BPD patient.
2. Moving through a consultative process and deciding whether to involve family.
3. Identifying appropriate level of care, treatment modality, and team roles.

Case Introduction

Susan is a 30-year-old woman who has a history of attachment difficulties as a child, suicidality since the age of 11, and anorexia nervosa during adolescence. In college, she struggled with symptoms of OCD, excessive shopping, and food addictions. Binge drinking began while in college in Boston. She has been in therapy since age 13, with one hospitalization at age 15 following an aborted suicide attempt. She has had multiple trials of antidepressants with little benefit while her drinking worsened. She has had principally psychodynamic treatments, though she had some exposure to DBT while in partial programming. Excessive drinking, multiple blackouts, and dangerous sexual involvements with men occurred frequently and potentiated her suicidal preoccupations. However, throughout her teens and twenties she completed college, worked in retail, and was accepted to law school though deferred her matriculation for a year.

When the initial call came to you requesting a treatment consultation, Susan was living in a sober house in Denver and had been sober for seven months, working part time in a restaurant. She had been having verbal outbursts and on one occasion had

---

J. Wheelis, M.D.
Department of Psychiatry, Harvard Medical School, McLean Hospital, Belmont, MA, USA
e-mail: jwheelis@partners.org

© Springer International Publishing AG, part of Springer Nature 2018
B. Palmer, B. Unruh (eds.), *Borderline Personality Disorder*,
https://doi.org/10.1007/978-3-319-90743-7_15

pushed a staff member. Her suicidality, irritability, and urges to drink were high. She was asked to leave the sober house.

The consultation request came from Susan's father, a prominent lawyer in Washington, DC. He received your name from one of Susan's former therapists who knew you from your psychiatry residency years in Boston, where you are now in private practice. Susan's current psychiatrist informs you that he recommended Susan suspend contact with her father as it had seemed to intensify her suicidal preoccupations.

Choice Point 1

For each intervention, choose H: "helpful," U: "unhelpful or harmful," or P: "perhaps helpful, with reservations."

With this information alone and thinking about initial steps for developing options for treatment, would you:

1. Recommend she seek inpatient psychiatric hospitalization nearby in Denver for further evaluation.
2. Set up a phone meeting with the father to discuss the situation.
3. Arrange for an in-person consultation with Susan.

Discussion

This is a complex consultation request as Susan is in Denver and you are in Boston. Yet even with limited information, you see that her instability in the sober house indicates a change in Susan's living and treatment arrangement is paramount. In your brief initial conversation with Susan's father, you ascertained that the family is willing to do whatever necessary to help their daughter but they are wary of exorbitant costs in view of their significant expenditure on treatment thus far. Coming east for treatment is potentially fraught as Susan attended college in Boston and during those years was highly agitated, suicidal, and drinking heavily.

Susan's suicidal ideation is concerning, but chronic. Mood instability is worrisome. In view of the fact that she is not drinking and there is no acute suicidality, an inpatient hospitalization is likely unnecessary and in the case of BPD is often harmful. Given the reported friction between Susan and her father, meeting with him initially, while useful with regards to collecting information, may limit the degree to which Susan could make an alliance with you as a therapist. An initial consultation face-to-face with Susan seems most prudent.

Answers

1. U
2. P
3. H

Principles and Clinical Pearls

1. Hospitalization, while often seeming convenient and containing, is frequently unnecessarily reinforcing maladaptive patterns of avoidance.
2. Family involvement is important, but it is important to frame the context and scope of this communication with the patient before proceeding.

Case Continues...

Susan arranges a consultation with you in Boston a week after your initial conversation with her father. She is anxious yet articulate, appealing, and intelligent. She describes her irritability as consistently high as well as her urges to drink. She complains of high suicidal ideation, impulsive spending and eating, and a sense of gloom about herself and her future. Her goals are to start law school, improve her relationship with her father, and make friends to feel more connected. She describes her relationship with her father as one she cannot stand having, and yet she simultaneously longs for it to be better. She tells you that her current psychiatrist feels that contact with her father will lead to acute suicide risk. She says she had been doing very well in a managerial position for a retail company in Denver. She feels at a loss as to what level of care and treatment modality would be appropriate for her as a next step.

Her past history is significant for being the eldest of four children. She was always good at school but suffered from marked social anxiety. She described her father as "loving, supportive, critical, terrifying, and unpredictable" and her mother as passive, funny, and deferential to her father. Her mother's pregnancy with her sister, the youngest of her siblings, precipitated the onset of Susan's suicidal preoccupation. Symptoms of OCD developed in middle school, including a multitude of rituals. She began drinking while away on a high-school year abroad. She came to Massachusetts for college where her binge drinking began. She recalled longing to die by alcohol poisoning. She was in therapy throughout college and then went to New York for 2 years during which time she had no therapy or contact with her father. She drank excessively and reported multiple dangerous situations with men while intoxicated. She had one aborted suicide attempt and her work performance in retail declined. She returned home to live with her parents and did volunteer work while studying for the LSAT exam and applying to law school. Her drinking and irritability increased and she then left home for residential treatment in Denver. She describes her mood instability as a 10 on a scale of 1–10.

Choice Point 2

At this point, would you:

1. Obtain consent to obtain her inpatient and partial hospital treatment records and to speak with her former therapists and psychopharmacologists.
2. Speak with her father and arrange for a family meeting.
3. Refer her to a residential or partial hospital program.

Discussion

The face-to-face meeting provides helpful additional information. Susan's history suggests intrapsychic conflict regarding her place in the family and the clear onset of difficulties associated with the birth of her youngest sibling. Inability to manage competitive strivings for parental care and special family roles (e.g., sole or favored daughter) frequently escalates BPD symptoms. Susan's intelligence and competence is significant yet it is unclear whether a high level of functioning is sustainable. Her drinking, overspending, overeating, and suicidal preoccupations are worrisome and suggest that emotion regulation is a significant and persistent concern. She is currently being treated with topiramate and clomipramine and a diagnosis of OCD has been noted along with depression, substance use disorder, and an eating disorder.

She has maintained performance at a job, yet this was in the context of a supervised sober living situation providing containment and support. Moving to Boston may be challenging in view of her past history of drinking while in college. However, she is confident she can easily transfer her job from Denver to Boston. Your assessment that she is able and committed to work part-time is essential for treatment planning, as ensuring sufficient structured activity external to the treatment will help her feel psychologically robust and have relevant real-world challenges to work productively in psychotherapy.

Obtaining records and speaking to prior treaters is extremely helpful at this point in the evaluation. The observations of others over time offer a window into previous clinical concerns about Susan as well as what she has, or has not, considered and learned in prior treatments.

A meeting with family will eventually be necessary to review your recommendations and ensure that the treatment is understandable and acceptable to all invested parties, but this may be premature as all the information is not yet available.

Residential treatment is a level of care worth considering, even though the father has mentioned cost as a significant consideration. Identifying appropriate resources and evaluating availability and cost is prudent at this stage. Partial hospital programming might be helpful as a transition. The alternative of setting up an outpatient treatment team is a challenge and requires that a primary therapy be identified along with adjunctive components including other individual and group services. Successful outpatient management of BPD requires close communication between all members of the identified treatment team.

Answers

1. H
2. P
3. P

Principles and Clinical Pearls

1. Determining the appropriate level of care requires careful assessment not just of symptoms and diagnosis, but of functioning over time and across a variety of settings. Such analysis requires consideration of observations and assessments made in past treatments. Obtaining records and speaking with former treaters is essential.

Case Continues...

Susan returns to Washington, DC, after your initial consultation, and you begin calling former therapists and obtaining old hospital records. Many of the former therapists express significant concern around irritability, isolation, and suicide risk while others more impressed by her intelligence, humor, and ability to relate genuinely in therapy are less preoccupied by safety concerns. It is noted that she has made good use of therapy and Alcoholics Anonymous while in Denver and particularly benefitted from the DBT components of treatment. Many therapists note that it has been hard to focus on many of the psychosocial determinants of her difficulties because of her worrisome behavior.

Her treatment records document longstanding questions about the possibility of bipolar illness. All psychopharmacological treatment has erred on treating the symptoms of depression and OCD, but with poor response. The current treaters are very worried about the toxicity of Susan's relationship with her father and feel that family involvement is not warranted. Several former therapists feel that there is a significant attachment problem in their relationship and that the mother has played a lesser more passive role to her father's assertive involvement. The former treaters are divided as to whether they believe Susan is able to manage an entirely outpatient treatment in the absence of a therapeutic milieu.

A call to a colleague at a residential treatment facility in Boston is reassuring as there is availability and a willingness to accept Susan if you recommend this level of care. The local partial hospital programs are full and the waitlist is several months out.

After two weeks of speaking with therapists and collecting past records, you are considering three possible treatment settings: (1) residential treatment for further evaluation and containment, which would involve treaters assigned by the program; (2) supervised living in a sober house with an outpatient treatment team; or (3) independent living in an apartment with an outpatient treatment team. The argument for residential or sober living level of care seems compelling given inconsistent functioning and sobriety during past outpatient treatments, but equally cogent is the notion that independent living seems critical for her goal to be in law school.

You arrange a conference call with Susan and her parents to review the options. In that call you learn that residential treatment is an unpopular option due to cost as well as its seeming "step backward" and Susan does not want to lose the autonomy about choosing her therapist. The sober house option is met with mixed feeling but a willingness to consider. Susan shares your concern that a more restrictive treatment arrangement would interfere with her ability to maintain her job and pursue longer-term vocational goals. Finally, while the call highlights the previously reported tension between Susan and her father, you also observe a lot of compatibility and similarity.

Within a few days, Susan calls and lets you know that she is most interested in putting together an outpatient team and living in a non-supervised apartment. You agree to be the primary therapist, provided that you and Susan can set up an acceptable plan for therapy that is financially viable.

Choice Point 3

At this point, would you:

1. Separate psychopharmacology from psychotherapy.
2. Establish DBT as the primary modality in Susan's treatment, recommending individual DBT and a DBT skills group.
3. Recommend adjunctive family therapy to address the problems in Susan's relationship with her father.
4. Recommend that Susan find a local Alchoholics Anonymous (AA) sponsor and attend AA meetings.
5. Recommend a case manager to help Susan and you oversee and coordinate components of care.
6. Insist on supervised sober living arrangement as a condition for therapy.

Discussion

In view of past records raising the question of bipolar disorder and your own appraisal of Susan's history of irritability, drinking, overspending, and promiscuity, there is ample reason to consider the possibility of this diagnosis. Careful psychopharmacological evaluation and monitoring is too significant an agenda to incorporate into her psychotherapy.

Susan specifically noted that DBT skills work was helpful in her recent treatment program. She has had multiple psychodynamic treatments with psychoanalysts in the past, which she feels were supportive and offered some insight about past conflicts but had limited scope of influence on her behavior. She feels her impulsive behavior and suicidality have frequently interfered with productive treatment. Individual DBT with use of a diary card would likely help her and you understand and organize her affective experiences and problematic behaviors in such a way as to help identify the specific problems to be solved.

In view of her conflictual familial relationships, it could be fruitful to have an adjunctive therapy specifically address those concerns. In view of the clear issues regarding attachment, use of the adult attachment interview and related treatment [1] might offer an organizing venue to address the profound problems noted in her relationship with her father.

Having a separate psychopharmacologist and an adjunctive family therapist now creates a team with multiple points of oversight in relation to Susan's progress. The question of session frequency remains. Standard individual DBT therapy is typically offered once and sometimes twice a week. Given that the treatment is aiming to help Susan start law school within a year's time and that the primary therapist will also be serving the function of a case manager, increased frequency seems appropriate. The adjunctive psychotherapy will commence at a lesser frequency as well as the psychopharmacology. The primary therapist should monitor all components of treatment via close communication with all treaters and reevaluate the optimal frequency of sessions over time.

AA involvement with a sponsor is important both for helping maintain sobriety but also as an antidote to Susan's chronic isolative tendencies. Learning DBT skills in the context of a group format rather than individually will have that added benefit as well. Susan has maintained close communication with sponsors and attended two to three AA meetings per week in the past. Supervised sober living would offer another point of oversight, containment, and social community. Yet Susan is disinclined to accept this and you share her wish that she have the opportunity to try independent living to evaluate her ability to manage in law school. Furthermore, she has just come from a supervised living situation in Denver in which she demonstrated a capacity to maintain employment and sobriety, but has yet to do so as an outpatient. You decide to focus the treatment on stabilizing her functional capacities as an outpatient.

In general, the function of case manager can be carved out from the primary therapist role. Yet in Susan's case, this would seem somewhat superfluous given that oversight of Susan's involvement in the designed treatment plan and close communication amongst the treaters will be essential to the primary therapist role. For patients with difficulty finding or maintaining a job or completing tasks of daily living, it can be more important to designate a separate, adjunctive case manager role.

You propose twice weekly individual DBT therapy, once weekly DBT skills group, once weekly adjunctive/family psychotherapy, and weekly psychopharmacology. Additionally, you recommend identifying a sponsor and attending 2–3 AA meetings each week. You propose monthly "family involvement" meetings with her parents to ensure her parents understand the treatment and how to be helpful and avoid contributing to unhelpful interventions. Finally, you recommend that the adjunctive therapist make recommendations for specific work on Susan's relationship with her father. You formalize a requirement for Susan to maintain at least 20 h of work per week as a contingency of remaining in treatment with you.

This treatment plan seems to target Susan's major areas of difficulties including affect regulation, impulsivity, attachment difficulties, social isolation, and difficulty generalizing gains made in residential treatment to outpatient settings. You review this treatment plan with Susan and her family and it is found acceptable by all.

Answers

1. H
2. H
3. H
4. H
5. P
6. P

Principles and Clinical Pearls

1. Outpatient BPD treatment planning should carefully designate the scope and aim of each proposed treatment component and role. The primary therapist is responsible for delivering the principal treatment modality and monitoring the patient's progress by overseeing all other components and coordinating with all involved treaters. Adjunctive treatments on multimodal BPD treatment teams typically include case management, psychopharmacology, family therapy, and group therapy, but a careful rationale for offering each element must be proposed.

Summary of Clinical Approach

Unlike other chapters, this chapter specifically addresses BPD treatment by specialists in the disorder, providing consultation for a complex case of a patient with considerable prior treatment experience but with limited overall benefit. Effective treatment planning for BPD patients begins with a consultant assessing the appropriate level of care by thoroughly evaluating current presenting problems as well as lessons learned, behavioral change sustained, and consistent functioning achieved – or the lack of these markers – across varying clinical settings and levels of support and containment. Reviewing collateral history and records from previous treatments is essential for comprehensive assessment. It is important to outline a level of care that supports the highest possible level of functioning without burdening patients beyond their capabilities. The consultant generally also determines the modality, scope, aim, and frequency of the primary therapy and each proposed adjunctive component, and assists with identifying clinicians to carry out each designated role. "Pre-treatment" meetings are usually held with prospective patients and their families, either jointly or separately, to outline the recommended treatment plan and obtain all parties' agreement to begin.

> **Clinician Experience: Tendency to Escalate Treatment Complexity on the Assumption that "More Is Better"**
> There is a tendency at times to believe that more treatment will always be helpful, especially where there is worry about suicidality, drinking, or other impulsive or risky behaviors. In fact, sometimes more treatment can be counterproductive, contributing to more passivity and less accountability on the part of both patients and clinicians. Adjunctive treatment components such as additional individual and group therapies and supervised or sober living situations can offer valuable additional support, but can also increase interpersonal tensions and problematic behaviors depending on how the patient's particular psychology interacts with the structural and interpersonal features of each component offered. Indiscriminately adding treatments can also foster a false sense of security that others are taking responsibility, when instead responsibility should be systematically localized within the primary clinician by formally delineating this role on the team and maintaining active coordination with and oversight of all treatment components.

Reference

1. Brown DP, Elliott DS, editors. Attachment disturbances in adults: treatment for comprehensive repair: WW Norton; New York; 2016.

Dr. Wheelis is an Assistant Clinical Professor of Psychiatry at Harvard Medical School and Associate Psychiatrist at McLean Hospital. She is the co-founder and director of Two Brattle Center, an outpatient mental health clinic in Cambridge, having served as clinical director since its inception in 1996. She began intensive training in Dialectical Behavior Therapy (DBT) in 1997 and became a DBT Trainer for Behavioral Tech in 2003. Additionally, she is a Training and Supervising Analyst at the Boston Psychoanalytic Society and Institute. Her expertise includes the treatment of suicidal patients and the development of intensive outpatient treatment programs as alternatives to hospital level clinical care.

Early Diagnosis and Intervention in Adolescents

16

Owen Muir and Carlene MacMillan

Choice Point Index
1. Establishing the treatment frame with previously undiagnosed youth and families
2. Addressing the comorbidity of borderline personality disorder (BPD) and post-traumatic stress disorder (PTSD) in youth
3. Understanding and explaining prior experiences with clinicians
4. The role of medications in adolescents with BPD
5. Management of suicidal threats and levels of care

Case Introduction

Luis is a 14-year-old boy of mixed Honduran and Caucasian ethnicity living with his parents and his brother in a neighborhood that has suffered significant storm damage from a major weather event 2 years ago. You are a resident working in a child psychiatric clinic when Luis is transferred to your care with a history of "depression and anxiety" and a recent diagnosis of attention deficit hyperactivity disorder (ADHD). He has a history of chronic suicidal ideation, high-risk sexual behaviors, poor school performance, truancy, and abuse of substances including alcohol, cannabis, cocaine, alprazolam, and more ("whatever I can get, really"). He also has a history of multiple traumatic experiences, including sexual trauma for which he is currently seeing a psychologist for evidence-based exposure-oriented treatment. Prior treatments include one prior psychiatric admission for a suicide

O. Muir, M.D. (✉)
Brooklyn Minds, Brooklyn, NY, USA
e-mail: owen.muir@brooklynminds.com

C. MacMillan, M.D.
Brooklyn Minds, Psychiatry, P.C. and Ellenhorn, L.L.C., New York, NY, USA

© Springer International Publishing AG, part of Springer Nature 2018
B. Palmer, B. Unruh (eds.), *Borderline Personality Disorder*,
https://doi.org/10.1007/978-3-319-90743-7_16

attempt, followed by a day treatment program offering skills groups and then 2 months of a specialized adolescent dialectical behavior therapy (DBT) program, which Luis claims was "useless" ("I know all the skills already").

Today Luis is meeting you for an initial session, having previously seen two trainees in the clinic for a year at a time. His medications include: sertraline 250 mg daily, quetiapine 200 mg nightly, lisdexamfetamine 70 mg daily, and clonazepam 0.5 mg as needed. His mother breaks down in tears as she accompanies him to your office from the waiting room and laments how difficult it has been living with "Hurricane Luis."

Choice Point 1

For each intervention, choose H: "helpful," U: "unhelpful or harmful," or P: "perhaps helpful, with reservations."

You ponder how best to establish a viable treatment frame, and whether additional information is needed before you can decide how to begin:

1. Extend the duration of the initial appointment beyond the usual 45 minutes allotted for a "transfer," to "retake the history," determine if Luis meets criteria for BPD, and allow time to discuss your impressions with the family.
2. Offer to see Luis monthly for medication management, as prior psychiatrists had done.
3. Refer him back to the DBT team to resume intensive outpatient DBT services and a "skills refresher."
4. Meet with Luis first without his mother, and promise you will keep his risky sexual behavior and substance use confidential from his mother.
5. Suggest that Luis meet with you weekly and refrain from making a diagnosis of BPD given Luis's age.

Discussion

One of the common difficulties in treating children and adolescents with a history of symptoms suggestive of BPD is the professional folklore that it cannot be diagnosed in an adolescent. This view is not supported by current diagnostic criteria in Section II of DSM-5, which states the diagnosis can be made in those under age 18 if symptoms have been persistent for greater than 1 year [1]. Section III of DSM-5, which outlines an alternate model for personality disorders, goes further by removing all duration criteria. Epidemiological data suggests that up to 3% of adolescents meet criteria for borderline personality disorder, including as many as 50% of psychiatrically hospitalized adolescents [2, 3].

Clinicians often find it challenging to distinguish many symptoms of BPD from typical teen behavior. However, while identity formation is a core component of adolescent development, most adolescents do not lack a core sense of self nor do they display severe emotional difficulties persistently. While experimentation with self-injury is relatively common, most do not chronically self-injure or attempt suicide to regulate their moods, or come to emergent psychiatric attention after a rift with a romantic partner or friend. Long-term epidemiological data suggests that, in retrospect, the average patient in a sample of adults that were hospitalized and subsequently diagnosed with BPD reports experiencing severe emotional difficulties before 11 years of age and self-injurious behavior beginning around age 12 [4]. A careful clinical assessment can tease apart typical adolescent behavior from behavior suggestive of BPD.

Yet, due to persistent stigma and misconceptions about BPD, the diagnosis is often either deliberately or unintentionally not made explicit in the adolescent population. This lost opportunity deprives patients and families of appropriate BPD-targeted early interventions [5]. Taking ample time on the first appointment to make an accurate diagnosis and provide psychoeducation around the course, prognosis, and appropriate treatments for BPD can help treatment begin on the right foot with a new patient and family. The extra time for careful history-taking and psychoeducation is especially important if past providers have given other diagnoses but did not identify BPD.

Although data are lacking for universal prevention efforts for BPD, "indicated prevention" in high risk youth and early intervention after the illness has appeared are approaches that hold promise for reducing the burden of BPD [6]. Indicated prevention would target the symptoms that often predict later development of PD in adolescents, such as disruptive behavior disorders [7, 8], depression [9, 10], and substance use disorders (especially alcohol use disorder) [11, 12]. Although deploying broadly effective treatment for at-risk youth with these other conditions is a significant undertaking, it does have the benefit of being the kind of collaborative work child and adolescent mental health providers are already likely more comfortable and well trained to do. Furthermore, these are significant illnesses to treat in their own right. Additionally, adaptations of existing therapies for BPD in adults such as DBT and mentalization-based treatment (MBT) appear to have promise both in theory [13, 14] and in randomized-controlled trials (RCTs) of DBT-C [15], [16] in disruptive behavior disorders.

Early intervention—treating BPD at the earliest presenting signs of the illness—is an approach that has already proven effective in other psychiatric disorders such as psychosis [17]. Early intervention in BPD is possible and preliminary trials have suggested there may be effective approaches [5, 6, 18]. Indeed, the predominant generalist BPD treatment model for adults has itself been proposed in an adapted form for the generalist treatment of youth with BPD [19, 20]. Furthermore, both DBT-A and mentalization-based treatment for adolescents (MBT-A) have been studied in adolescents presenting with self-injury as a presenting complaint with promising results in randomized controlled trials [21–23].

In terms of evaluating possible responses to this choice point, although continuing monthly medication management visits is possibly helpful, the GPM recommendation is to have weekly visits if feasible. This case already involves a psychologist working weekly with the patient, and this may be sufficient with regular communication between providers.

In terms of a referral back to the DBT-A team, in this case the patient has already demonstrated a lack of meaningful adherence to that treatment model, which, although frequently effective, requires substantial commitment on the part of patients and families to receive maximum benefit. Sometimes, the knee-jerk reaction to seeing an individual with BPD is to say "they need DBT!" and while immensely valuable for many, for some patients there will be diminishing returns and alternate approaches should be considered.

When working with adolescent patients with personality disorders, the dilemma of balancing a desire to maintain confidentiality regarding risky behaviors while at the same time recognizing the reality that a minor has legal guardians who need to have some idea of the risks involved comes up frequently. Openly presenting this dilemma to the adolescent and working collaboratively to find an effective way to share information on a "need to know" basis with caretakers is an important aspect of building a functional alliance with an adolescent who may be quite mistrustful at baseline. For example, occasional marijuana smoking may not need to be disclosed but use of heroin is a very different level of risk that generally cannot be kept a secret.

When thinking of weekly treatment with Luis, it is worth considering if this will likely benefit Luis in terms of "extending the evaluation" as well as providing the chance for ongoing psychoeducation and GPM-informed care. However, given that Luis is already in individual therapy, it is worth considering the role of family involvement in the case as opposed to more individual work, given the mother's level of distress as well.

Answers

1. H
2. P
3. U
4. U
5. U

Principles and Clinical Pearls

1. BPD is a diagnosis that can and should be made in adolescence when it is appropriate and should not be delayed until an individual turns 18.
2. Ensuring diagnostic accuracy, providing psychoeducation, and being available to answer questions is the best way to make sure patients and families benefit from hearing the BPD diagnosis. A well-delivered explanation of BPD's diagnostic features, etiology, available treatments, and typical course is almost universally experienced as validating and helpful. When possible, it is worth scheduling extra time to ensure treatment starts with establishing a shared understanding and your trustworthiness as a knowledgeable and helpful guide.

3. Specialized treatments like DBT-A and MBT-A have proven efficacy in the treatment of BPD, but they are not a good fit for all patients and are not widely accessible in many places. A well-informed generalist approach can be effective, especially for patients who are not interested in specialized treatment or have already had an unhelpful trial of one or more of them.

Case Continues...

Your extended initial evaluation shows Luis meets all nine criteria for BPD and full criteria for PTSD due to a sexual assault he suffered while intoxicated. You find your initial meeting with both the patient and his mother to be enjoyable, and sense they feel supported by and connected with you. When Luis is alone with you, he is quite open, even surprisingly frank about his difficulties, but once you bring his mother into the room the dynamic changes. The emotional temperature of the room rises to levels where it is hard to think clearly. Luis and his mom hurl accusations at each other, thwarting your initial efforts to support them both by explaining your diagnosis and proposed treatment plan. His mother exclaims frantically, "He says he's traumatized, but I am traumatized by him! Maybe we all have PTSD!" You consider how best to move forward with both Luis and his mother, given the volatility between them. You also want to address the interplay of BPD and PTSD.

Choice Point 2

You consider how best to address the comorbidity of BPD and PTSD:

1. Express your agreement with the PTSD diagnosis and explain that BPD is essentially another way to explain trauma, so nothing is gained by saying Luis has both BPD and PTSD.
2. Tell Luis and his mother that your treatment will focus on PTSD, and postpone introducing the BPD diagnosis until achieving a better alliance with Luis' mother.
3. Schedule separate psychoeducation sessions for Luis and for his parents, in which you will present both BPD and PTSD diagnoses and their interaction, emphasizing BPD as primary focus for treatment now.
4. Call Luis' current therapist (a trauma specialist using a trauma-focused cognitive behavioral therapy (CBT) protocol) to obtain collateral history before discussing your diagnostic impression and treatment recommendations.
5. Meet separately with Luis' mother to validate her difficulties and educate her about the transactional nature of BPD-related problems, including guidelines for ways she can respond more effectively to Luis.

Discussion

Providing psychoeducation for adolescents with newly diagnosed BPD and their families is crucial. For many, this may be the first time the diagnosis has even been suggested. Providing enough time at treatment outset for both patients and families to absorb information and to ask questions is beneficial. If the relational dynamics within the family system seem too volatile, it is preferable to schedule separate appointments to explain the diagnosis rather than insist on tackling the family dynamic right away.

While most patients with BPD report longstanding experiences of feeling invalidated, neglected, or misunderstood, the role of discrete trauma in the etiology of BPD has been historically overvalued. Some clinicians incorrectly conclude that adding a BPD diagnosis for patients who clearly meet criteria for PTSD is unnecessary and unhelpful. However, factor analysis studies of BPD's variance have since shown that only 15% is explained by traumatic experiences, while over 55% relates to genetic factors [24]. While important to not overlook patients' descriptions of their lives as "traumatizing," it would be inaccurate and harmful to withhold a BPD diagnosis when criteria are met simply because you want to take seriously a report of "trauma." BPD and PTSD have only partially overlapping evidence-based treatments, for example. Some psychotherapies that are effective for PTSD (e.g., trauma-focused cognitive behavioral therapy (TF-EMDR), eye movement desensitization and reprograming (EMDR)) are rendered less effective when BPD is present, whereas others (e.g., prolonged exposure, DBT-PTSD) retain effectiveness in the context of comorbid BPD [25]. Thus, it is important to speak with Luis' trauma therapist to ascertain whether the trauma treatment being delivered is one that could be expected to help in the context of comorbid BPD and PTSD, at the same time as you are intending to begin BPD-targeted treatment.

One way to highlight the relationship between BPD and traumatic invalidation (as opposed to discrete, episodic traumatic events) is to explain how recurrent invalidating experiences foster an entrenched mistrust in close relationships, toward purported authorities, and about new social learning from any source [26]. Identifying mistrust as a common result of recurrent invalidation establishes a helpful shared understanding you can return to later in treatment when mistrust arises. It can be helpful to ask, "might your difficulties with trust be relevant to what is happening right now (with me … with your friends … with your parents)?" When explaining feelings of invalidation, it is also important to point out to caretakers that this can happen even when a caretaker has made significant efforts to support the adolescent. Learning ways to more effectively validate someone with BPD is often a core component of the family work, as validation can sometimes be quite counter-intuitive.

Answers

1. U
2. U
3. H
4. P
5. H

Principles and Clinical Pearls

1. Accurate assessment of comorbidities is essential. While many comorbidities should be considered secondary to initiating BPD treatment, some are priority treatment targets in their own right and should be managed concurrently (such as PTSD) or before treating BPD (bipolar I when actively manic, active substance dependence).
2. BPD and PTSD are separate diagnostic entities, despite common assertions that they are different lenses through which to approach the same set of problems.
3. Emphasizing to caregivers that validation is often counter-intuitive for individuals with BPD and that a young person feeling invalidated does not mean they did a "bad job" raising their child.

Case Continues...

You meet with Luis alone for a second time to explain the BPD diagnosis at length and ensure he understands you will be initiating treatment for BPD at the same time as he completes his final prolonged exposure sessions for PTSD. Luis replied, in a jocular tone, "Yeah, I looked up BPD when they put me in DBT. That's what DBT was invented for. I totally have that! Why did everyone just keep saying I had depression and anxiety? Why hasn't my therapist told me about this?"

Choice Point 3

How would you respond to Luis's questions?

1. "I don't know why this diagnosis wasn't made earlier" (said in a neutral, unemotional tone).
2. "I don't know why this diagnosis wasn't made earlier. A lot of people miss it. Seems like that is annoying to you? Honestly, I think the diagnosis should be made more readily.
3. "It's possible that since symptoms and people change over time, different doctors might have been right at different points in time."
4. "Some doctors just don't ask the right questions."
5. "Some clinicians aren't aware that BPD is treatable, and that can influence their willingness to give what they might understand as bad news."

Discussion

In an under-diagnosed condition like BPD, it is common for adolescents to have seen a number of providers and have received other less accurate diagnoses before getting a definitive BPD diagnosis. Even adolescent patients treated in formal DBT programs do not always receive the diagnosis despite meeting criteria. Sometimes clinicians will make the diagnosis "behind the scenes" when discussing cases in supervision but will refrain from informing the adolescent and their family. While understandably frustrating for patients and families, this scenario provides the savvy clinician an opportunity to employ a "not-knowing" stance around the perspectives and decision-making of others. This is challenging for patients with BPD who are prone to non-nuanced, overly certain, black-and-white judgments about others and have difficulty exploring a variety of perspectives about others' thoughts, feelings, and actions toward them. A shared aim of several empirically validated treatments for BPD in adolescence is to foster greater awareness that multiple alternate perspectives are possible in a given situation. It would be harmful to "throw under the bus" Luis' previous clinicians, as this would miss an opportunity to model reckoning with alternate viewpoints and curiosity needed to consider how discrepant diagnoses might have come about. Some display of emotion, if genuine and "contingent" (in keeping with what patients themselves are likely feeling)—can help patients feel more trust in your involvement as an authentic person who cares. Being "a real person" with your own set of thoughts and feelings that you are willing to judiciously convey as your own (not assumed to be identical to your patients' experiences) can help adolescents with a poor sense of self maintain a sense of both differentiation from and connection with you.

Answers

1. P
2. H
3. P
4. U
5. H

Principles and Clinical Pearls

1. Demonstrating a sense of non-judgmental and authentic curiosity about the experiences an adolescent has had with prior clinicians helps model appropriate perspective-taking and reflection.
2. Displaying appropriately modulated but genuine emotional reactions of your own can help build trust with mistrustful patients who struggle to accurately interpret more affectively detached, neutral clinical responses.

Case Continues...

On the next visit Luis returns with his mother, who explains, "We have been reading a lot about this BPD thing, and it makes so much sense! But we read there is no medication for BPD! How are you going to help him?" Luis adds, "Well, my best friend's "Xanny bar" helps ... can I get some of that? At least give me something to feel a little better!"

Choice Point 4

How would you respond to Luis and his mother's questions?

1. Prescribe alprazolam 0.5 mg, four times daily as needed for anxiety.
2. State you will continue his prescription for clonazepam, explaining it works similarly but is less addictive.
3. Decline alprazolam and, assuming the patient had been taking clonazepam sparingly, make a plan to taper and eventually discontinue it.
4. Screen for any other substances Luis may have used, misused, or abused to find relief.
5. Emphasize that psychosocial interventions comprise the main treatment for BPD, and medications should play at best a secondary role.
6. Convert his quetiapine dose to extended-release quetiapine 150 mg daily to fit the dose shown effective for treating BPD-related impulsivity in a published randomized controlled trial in adults.

Discussion

The role of pharmacotherapies in treating BPD in adolescents who are especially susceptible to adverse metabolic effects of antipsychotic medications [27] should be limited to the management of comorbidities. There are no FDA-approved medications for BPD in any age group, and the one "positive" trial of extended-release quetiapine extended release [28] had numerous methodological problems in its adult sample, calling into question the already limited applicability for adolescents with BPD. Managing comorbidities, however, is indicated, so medications might be considered for Luis' comorbid symptoms including inattention and hyperactivity/impulsivity related to ADHD (e.g., stimulants and alpha-agonists) and sleep disturbance and nightmares related to PTSD (e.g., prazosin).

It can be tempting in highly behaviorally distressed adolescents to prescribe antipsychotics. However, in adolescents with BPD without comorbid bipolar disorder or psychotic illnesses, antipsychotic use is highly discouraged. Even theoretically "lower-risk" antipsychotic medications like aripiprazole have definitive associations with significant metabolic adverse effects in children including diabetes, dyslipidemia, and bone density abnormalities [29–31]. Sometimes clinicians will prescribe lamotrigine as a mood stabilizer since it is generally well tolerated and there may be a perception that it "cannot hurt." However, the risk of Stevens–Johnson syndrome, a potentially fatal rash, is thought to be higher in the pediatric population [32]. The risk/benefit ratio makes it hard to justify its routine usage for BPD in adolescents. It is better to provide a rationale for tapering down or discontinuing any medications that have not demonstrated significant effectiveness for the patient. Explanations for why "less is more" are part of a larger goal of reducing iatrogenic harm. Thoughtful "de-prescribing" is also consistent with the expectation for natural improvement over time.

Longitudinal data around the use of benzodiazepines in patients with BPD suggests that these medications exacerbate the course of illness [33, 34]. The risks of benzodiazepines for these patients are amply documented, including the risk of dependence and life-threatening withdrawal. Alprazolam is particularly problematic with its high lipophilicity and short half-life lending a similarity to the pharmacokinetic and absorption profile of most drugs of abuse. It has significant street value because it can provide a significant "high." Furthermore, its short half-life multiple times a day, the pernicious belief that medications are an appropriate, or even the best, treatment for the interpersonal is driving core emotional difficulties in BPD. Substance use disorders are common in BPD, and even more so during adolescence. Inquiry about substance use, misuse, and diversion is always appropriate, and should be addressed with evidence-based interventions. Although treatment of severe substance use disorders in adolescence entails the use of specialized skills, it is incumbent on those who treat adolescents with BPD to either acquire such skills themselves or work collaboratively with addiction specialists to ensure best possible outcomes in all domains.

Prescribing is sometimes helpful for alliance-building when patients or families seek a concrete display of support. A relatively less harmful approach is to offer a selective serotonin reuptake inhibitor (SSRI) in some cases, as this category of medication has shown some limited efficacy for certain BPD symptoms. As you do so, you should insist that desired outcomes for the prescription are clearly identified and collaboratively tracked with input from patients as well as families, and that medications are regarded as adjuncts while psychosocial interventions such as individual and group therapies are prioritized [24]. However, antidepressants carry a black-box warning in the pediatric population for potentially increasing suicidal ideation so even a trial of a commonly prescribed SSRI is not without its risk and should involve close monitoring and psychoeducation.

Answers

1. U
2. U
3. H
4. H
5. H
6. U

Principles and Clinical Pearls

1. "Skills, not pills": aggressive prescribing is relatively contraindicated in all BPD treatment, but especially for adolescents who are at higher risk of both predictable

and unpredictable iatrogenic harms of medications. Emphasize learning behavioral skills and perspective-taking as effective approaches for managing emotional dysregulation, and limit iatrogenic harm with systematic de-prescribing.

2. Assess substance use disorders: caring for adolescents with borderline personality disorder inherently requires diligence in the assessment of substance use disorders, and appropriate treatment or referral to appropriate treatment for substance use disorders, without which progress in treatment is unlikely to be made.

Case Continues...

Luis does not return to school after winter break, having met a new love interest while on a ski trip. He says that school makes him feel suicidal because the teachers all have it out for him and the kids are bullies. His mom has taken away his privileges to play video games, but this has not made a difference. You are called by the ER psychiatric resident after Luis has self-injured in the context of his mom taking away his cell phone for refusing to go to school and "sexting" with his new girlfriend. He says he is suicidal and wants to go to the hospital but his mother says he just wants to avoid going back to school. You are contemplating what to recommend.

Choice Point 5

What will you say to the ER resident?

1. Since he has expressed suicidal ideation and self-injured, and has been refusing to go to school, recommend he be admitted to a locked inpatient psychiatric facility.
2. Recommend he remain in the ER at least until the morning, potentially in an observation bed, and arrange to speak with him and his mother in the morning to get a better sense of what might be helpful at this time.
3. Recommend that his parents hire an educational consultant to begin looking at alternative placements such as therapeutic boarding schools, wilderness programs, and online schools.
4. Obtain permission to speak to his school counselor, and work with the school and his therapist to ensure he has appropriate support at school and arrange a plan for him to gradually return.

Discussion

Hospitalization of adolescents with BPD should not be undertaken lightly and can often cause more unintended harm than good. For adolescents, attendance at school is effectively their "job." Hospitalization for someone already refusing to attend school increases the degree to which they fall behind academically and socially [35]. Brief acute hospitalization is generally reserved for when an adolescent has comorbid conditions requiring intensive treatment in a monitored medical setting (e.g., mania warranting rapid loading of a mood stabilizer), or when the adolescent's living situation and support network are too unstable to manage a crisis involving acute threats of suicide or harm to others. In Luis's case, both he and his mother seem open to working in the outpatient setting so it is likely a hospitalization would be more of a setback than of benefit. However, statements about suicide do warrant careful assessment.

Sometimes in the immediate aftermath of a fight with a key attachment figure, such as a parent, thorough safety assessment is nearly impossible. In these cases, many emergency rooms are able to place individuals on a time-limited observational status until the affective temperature cools down enough to perform a careful assessment. During that time, caregivers should be encouraged to leave the adolescent in the care of the emergency room staff overnight. Remaining at the bedside can unintentionally amplify suicidal statements, as caregivers' attention to the adolescent is naturally heightened in these crises [36].

When emotions have cooled enough to devise an effective plan, it can be tempting in the aftermath of a crisis to recommend extreme measures such as wilderness programs, therapeutic boarding schools, and other alternative settings. Before exploring these options, caregivers can often work with the adolescent's school to craft a plan to reintroduce the school environment thoughtfully. Psychiatrists and other mental health professionals have an active role to play in providing guidance to families and school staff on best practices for returning. Individual education plans (IEPs) are not only for learning differences but can also be developed to assist an individual with BPD and suicidal ideation and school refusal in transitioning back to school [37]. If the adolescent's attempts to return to school go poorly and it becomes clear to all involved that it is not working despite reasonable interventions having been tried, school districts are then in the position of providing funds toward alternative placements such as therapeutic schools, which can be quite costly. The spectrum of alternatives is broad and due diligence is needed to appropriately vet the programs being considered [38]. Educational consultants have expertise in this area. Families should ask programs about what evidence-based practices they use, outcomes, and level of staff experience in working with adolescents with BPD.

Answers

1. U
2. P
3. P
4. H

Principles and Clinical Pearls

1. Although suicidal threats and other concerning behaviors such as frequent school refusal warrant careful assessment, reflex hospitalization can be harmful.

2. Psychiatrists and other mental health professionals working with adolescents with BPD have an active role to play in collaborating with school systems to address BPD symptoms that get in the way of the adolescent achieving success at school.

Summary of Clinical Approach

Most patients with BPD experience symptoms beginning in childhood, with onset of self-injury most often before the teenage years. Understanding BPD in adolescents should therefore be considered a core competency in child and adolescent mental health care. Accurate recognition and disclosure of the diagnosis is crucial to the treatment of BPD in adolescence. This should be followed by thorough psychoeducation for patients, families, and other involved mental health and medical professionals to counter erroneous and stigmatized conceptualizations of the disorder. Psychoeducation should be grounded in a developmental context distinguishing clear signs of BPD from normative adolescent behavior. It is important to highlight the transactional nature of factors in the home that can perpetuate or exacerbate BPD's course so that parents can seek effective coaching and support as well.

Treatment plans should prioritize BPD unless any comorbidity is deemed primary. Effective treatment for BPD requires effective assessment of co-occurring conditions, which include substance use disorders. Assessment for the presence or development of substance use disorders should be routine.

As is the case in adults with BPD, psychotherapy is the first-line intervention for adolescents with BPD. There are significant effect sizes in randomized controlled trials for adaptations of two major approaches proven effective for adults, DBT and MBT. In this regard, BPD is in keeping with the growing body of evidence suggesting that psychotherapy is often superior to pharmacotherapy for most conditions of childhood (with Attention Deficit/Hyperactivity Disorder as a notable exception) [39, 40]. Pharmacological treatment should ideally be limited to managing co-occurring conditions per evidence-based algorithms. Particular caution should be given in prescribing medications for acute agitation, as long-term use poses significant metabolic harm over time (antipsychotics, mood stabilizers) or addictive and diversion potential (benzodiazepines). Hospitalization for symptoms of BPD in adolescents should play a very limited role, if any. Interventions to help the adolescent thrive in their home and school environment should be emphasized.

This chapter has applied core principles of Good Psychiatric Management (GPM) to the care of adolescents presenting with BPD. Although GPM was not studied as a model in an adolescent population, GPM's principles closely resemble those of "good enough" children and adolescent psychiatry. However, due to the national shortage of child psychiatrists, many adult psychiatrists are tasked with taking care of these adolescents. Furthermore, even many child and adolescent psychiatrists feel ill-equipped to manage adolescents presenting with BPD, as this area is often overlooked during child/adolescent fellowship training. The GPM treatment manual is a recommended orienting device for clinicians of any training background caring for adolescents with BPD.

Clinician Experience: Getting Through to Mistrustful Adolescents Through "Radical Genuineness," Transparency, and "Marking"

Adolescents with BPD struggle even more than their healthy peers or adult BPD counterparts to accurately process the intentions and attitudes underlying the visible aspects of interpersonal relationships (e.g., facial expression, tone of voice, and what is done or not done). Unclear and emotionally distant communications by clinicians are likely to be interpreted unreflectively through a pervasive lens of mistrust, providing fuel to negative expectations of relationships that can easily undermine treatment alliance early on.

Trust can be facilitated over time through high levels of self-disclosure and of what DBT labels as "radical genuineness" and what MBT labels as "marking." Transparently expressing your own thoughts and feelings with respect to your patients, and "marking" them as your own fallible assessment helps put adolescent patients at greater ease during clinical encounters by reducing mystery, demonstrating emotional involvement, and inviting them to clarify points of potential misunderstanding. Your professional stance should be one of genuinely and clearly communicating your own thoughts and feelings as well as your grasp of how your patient responds. When in doubt about what to say next, fall back on "curious, connected, and caring" language with an attention to the tone of voice and body language.

References

1. American Psychiatric Association. Borderline personality disorder. Diagnostic and statistical manual of mental disorders. 5th ed. Arlington: American Psychiatric Publishing; 2013. p. 663–6.
2. Bernstein DP, Cohen P, Velez CN, Schwab-Stone M, Siever LJ, Shinsato L. Prevalence and stability of the DSM-III-R personality disorders in a community-based survey of adolescents. Am J Psychiatry. 1993;150:1237–43.
3. Moran P, Coffey C, Mann A, Carlin JB, Patton GC. Personality and substance use disorders in young adults. Br J Psychiatry. 2006;188:374–9.
4. Zanarini MC, Frankenburg FR, Ridolfi ME, Jager-Hyman S, Hennen J, Gunderson JG. Reported childhood onset of self-mutilation among borderline patients. J Personal Disord. 2006;20(1):9–15.
5. Chanen AM, Jackson HJ, McCutcheon LK, Jovev M, Dudgeon P, Yuen HP, Germano D, Nistico H, McDougall E, Weinstein C, Clarkson V, McGorry PD. Early intervention for adolescents with borderline personality disorder using cognitive analytic therapy: randomised controlled trial. Br J Psychiatry. 2008a;193.6:477–84.
6. Chanen AM, et al. Borderline personality disorder in young people and the prospects for prevention and early intervention. Curr Psychiatr Rev. 2008b;4(1):48–57.
7. Bernstein DP, Cohen P, Skodol A, Bezirganian S, Brook J. Childhood antecedents of adolescent personality disorders. Am J Psychiatry. 1996;153:907–13.
8. Zoccolillo M, Pickles A, Quinton D, Rutter M. The outcome of childhood conduct disorder: implications for defining adult person- ality disorder and conduct disorder. Psychol Med. 1992;22:971–86.

9. Cohen P, Crawford TN, Johnson JG, Kasen S. The children in the community study of developmental course of personality disorder. J Personal Disord. 2005;19:466–86.
10. Lewinsohn PM, Rohde P, Seeley JR, Klein DN. Axis II psychopathology as a function of Axis I disorders in childhood and adolescence. J Am Acad Child Adolesc Psychiatry. 1997;36:1752–9.
11. Rohde P, Lewinsohn PM, Kahler CW, Seeley JR, Brown RA. Natural course of alcohol use disorders from adolescence to young adulthood. J Am Acad Child Adolesc Psychiatry. 2001;40:83–90.
12. Thatcher DL, Cornelius JR, Clark DB. Adolescent alcohol use disorders predict adult borderline personality. Addict Behav. 2005;30:1709–24.
13. Perepletchikova F, Goodman G. Two approaches to treating preadolescent children with severe emotional and behavioral problems: dialectical behavior therapy adapted for children and mentalization-based child therapy. J Psychother Integr. 2014;24(4):298.
14. Midgley N, et al. Mentalization-based treatment for children: a time-limited approach: American Psychological Association; Washington, DC. 2017. http://www.apa.org/pubs/books/4317444.aspx.
15. Perepletchikova F, Nathanson D, Axelro, SR, Merrill C, Walker A, Grossman M, Mauer E. Randomized clinical trial of dialectical behavior therapy for preadolescent children with disruptive mood dysregulation disorder: feasibility and outcomes. J Am Acad Child Adolesc Psychiatry. 2017;56(10):832–40.
16. MacMillan C, Hassuk B. Confidently approaching borderline personality disorder in young people: a primer for the general child and adolescent psychiatrist. J Am Acad Child Adolesc Psychiatry. 2016;55(10):S17.
17. Kane JM, et al. Comprehensive versus usual community care for first-episode psychosis: 2-year outcomes from the NIMH RAISE early treatment program. Am J Psychiatry. 2015;173.4:362–72.
18. Chanen AM, McCutcheon L. Prevention and early intervention for borderline personality disorder: current status and recent evidence. Br J Psychiatry. 2013;202(s54):s24–9.
19. Muir OS. 24.1 Good Psychiatric Management (GPM) for personality disorders in young people. J Am Acad Child Adolesc Psychiatry. 2017;56(10):S35.
20. MacMillan C, Hassuk B. 24.0 personality disorders in young people: a primer for the generalist. J Am Acad Child Adolesc Psychiatry. 2017;56.10:S35.
21. Fleischhaker C, et al. Dialectical behavioral therapy for adolescents (DBT-A): a clinical trial for patients with suicidal and self-injurious behavior and borderline symptoms with a one-year follow-up. Child Adolesc Psychiatr Ment Health. 2011;5(1):3.
22. Mehlum L, et al. Dialectical behavior therapy for adolescents with repeated suicidal and self-harming behavior: a randomized trial. J Am Acad Child Adolesc Psychiatry. 2014;53(10):1082–91.
23. Rossouw TI, Fonagy P. Mentalization-based treatment for self-harm in adolescents: a randomized controlled trial. J Am Acad Child Adolesc Psychiatry. 2012;51(12):1304–13.
24. Gunderson JG. Handbook of good psychiatric management for borderline personality disorder: American Psychiatric Pub; 2014. p. 23.
25. Steil R, et al. DBT-PTSD. Trauma und Gewalt. 2010;4.2:106–17.
26. Fonagy P, Allison E. The role of mentalizing and epistemic trust in the therapeutic relationship. Psychotherapy. 2014;51(3):372.
27. Correll CU, Lencz T, Malhotra AK. Antipsychotic drugs and obesity. Trends Mol Med. 2011;17(2):97–107.
28. Black DW, et al. Comparison of low and moderate dosages of extended-release quetiapine in borderline personality disorder: a randomized, double-blind, placebo-controlled trial. Am J Psychiatr. 2014;171(11):1174–82.
29. Correll C, et al. Dysglycemic signals in children and adolescents treated with antipsychotics for the first time. Schizophr Res. 2014;153:S19.
30. Correll CU, et al. Effects of antipsychotics, antidepressants and mood stabilizers on risk for physical diseases in people with schizophrenia, depression and bipolar disorder. World Psychiatry. 2015;14(2):119–36.

31. Margari L, et al. Tolerability and safety profile of risperidone in a sample of children and adolescents. Int Clin Psychopharmacol. 2013;28.4:177–83.
32. Messenheimer JA. Rash in adult and pediatric patients treated with lamotrigine. Can J Neurol Sci. 1998;25(S4):S14–8.
33. Abraham PF, Calabrese JR. Evidenced-based pharmacologic treatment of borderline personality disorder: a shift from SSRIs to anticonvulsants and atypical antipsychotics? J Affect Disord. 2008;111:21–30.
34. Soloff PH. Psychopharmacology of borderline personality disorder. Psychiatr Clin N Am. 2000;23:169–92.
35. Preyde M, Parekh S, Heintzman J. Youths' experiences of school re-integration following psychiatric hospitalization. J Can Acad Child Adolesc Psychiatry. 2018;27(1):22.
36. Paris J. Is hospitalization useful for suicidal patients with borderline personality disorder? J Personal Disord. 2004;18(3):240.
37. Maynard BR, et al. Treatment for school refusal among children and adolescents: a systematic review and meta-analysis. Res Soc Work Pract. 2018;28(1):56–67.
38. Scott DA, Duerson LM. Continuing the discussion: a commentary on "Wilderness therapy: ethical considerations for mental health professionals". Child Youth Care Forum. 2010;39(1. Springer US):63.
39. Watson HJ, Rees CS. Meta-analysis of randomized, controlled treatment trials for pediatric obsessive-compulsive disorder. J Child Psychol Psychiatry. 2008;49(5):489–98.
40. Walkup JT, et al. Cognitive behavioral therapy, sertraline, or a combination in childhood anxiety. N Engl J Med. 2008;359(26):2753–66.

Dr. Muir is a child and adolescent psychiatrist on staff at Rockland Children's Psychiatric Center, a state hospital in New York, as well as the Medical Director of Brooklyn Minds, a group mental health practice in Brooklyn, NY. He is a graduate of The University of Rochester School of Medicine and Dentistry, completed residency at The Zucker Hillside Hospital, and completed Child and Adolescent Psychiatry fellowship training at the NYU School of Medicine.

Dr. MacMillan is a child and adolescent psychiatrist and the Medical Director of the NYC branch of Ellenhorn, a Private Assertive Community Treatment team. She is also the Clinical Director at Brooklyn Minds. Dr. MacMillan graduated from Harvard Medical School, and completed general and child/adolescent psychiatry training at Massachusetts General Hospital and McLean Hospital. Both are committed to the improvement in the care and diagnosis of youth with complex disorders of the self and participate in research, training, and advocacy at a local, national, and international level related to care of complex and "hard to reach" youth.

When Less May Be More: Scaling Limited Treatment Resources Using a Stepped-Care Model

Daniel Price

Choice Point Index
1. Making the diagnosis and initiating a treatment with hopefulness
2. Expecting accountability and engendering collaboration in evaluating treatment effectiveness
3. Managing priorities in the presence of comorbid substance use
4. Responding pragmatically when individual treatment is not sufficient
5. Managing resources when treatment is not progressing

Case Introduction

Lily is a 30-year-old woman being treated by Sarah, a PGY3 psychiatric resident in your department's training program. You are the expert in personality disorders, and Sarah has asked for your advice about treating Lily, who first evaluated Sarah a few weeks ago in the emergency department (ED), where she is well-known for repeatedly presenting intoxicated and suicidal. This time she was brought in by ambulance after a friend called 911 upon seeing that Lily had posted onto social media a picture of herself cutting with the caption: "the first cut is the deepest." In the ED Lily was disheveled, smelled of alcohol, and had a blood alcohol content of 0.25. She was initially combative and received an injection of an atypical antipsychotic after repeatedly banging on the ED door window threatening to break it down. She eventually slept, allowing examination of a 5 cm laceration on her forearm that ultimately required six sutures. She awoke early the next morning with little memory of the night before, and was at this point evaluated by Sarah in a holding room.

D. Price, M.D.
Department of Psychiatry, Maine Medical Center, Tufts University School of Medicine, Portland, ME, USA
e-mail: priced@mmc.org

© Springer International Publishing AG, part of Springer Nature 2018
B. Palmer, B. Unruh (eds.), *Borderline Personality Disorder*,
https://doi.org/10.1007/978-3-319-90743-7_17

Sarah initially found Lily angry, irritable, and a little scary. At first Lily lay on the gurney with the covers pulled up over her head, not speaking. With some persistence, Sarah was able to establish some rapport allowing for an informative interview. Having heard your didactic on borderline personality disorder (BPD) earlier in the year, she remembered that self-injurious behaviors often follow interpersonal stress and probed specifically whether anyone had let her down last night. Lily explained that after learning her boyfriend was cheating on her, she drank one fifth of a gallon of coffee brandy, took "a few oxy's," and made angry and disorganized posts on Facebook. At some point she cut herself and felt some relief. Lily believed she had become rapidly depressed on learning about her boyfriend's infidelity, saying, "My bipolar just does that." Lily said she was no longer suicidal and did not want to be hospitalized, because of a difficult admission when she was 19 that involved her being put into restraints. Sarah instead recommended Lily begin in a partial hospital program affiliated with your department. Lily made no promise to show up, but agreed to the plan while saying that Sarah was the first doctor who had "really listened."

Lily's course at the partial program was rocky. She was unhappy with being required to attend all the groups, arguing "I just don't do groups." During the second week, she came to the morning check-in group evidently intoxicated. She was asked to go home and return once she was sober. She angrily denied she was intoxicated at the time, but left and did not return for a few days. The program staff explored her alcohol use, and Lily quipped, "I don't have a problem with alcohol ... I have a problem *without* alcohol ... it's called bipolar disorder." She went on to say that she is treating her moods with alcohol, and it is the only thing that makes her feel better.

Lily stabilized somewhat after 2 weeks in the partial program, no longer making suicidal statements and reporting she had not cut during her stay. She began attending groups, though declined to participate. She was referred for outpatient follow-up, and because she remembers really liking "that student doctor," program staff contacted Sarah to ask if she would be willing to work with Lily. Sarah is now coming to you for advice about this. She wants to take Lily on, and sees herself working with patients like her, but expresses some worries: "I'm just starting in therapy, and Lily seems very ill. I worry she needs an expert or she won't get better, and I am far from an expert, especially in BPD."

Choice Point 1

For each intervention, choose H: "helpful," U: "unhelpful or harmful," or P: "perhaps helpful, with reservations."

In response to Lily's concerns, you:

1. Agree and say that Sarah needs more training before beginning with a patient like Lily.
2. Agree, saying Lily needs a specialized treatment and as Sarah is not trained in dialectical behavior therapy (DBT) or mentalization-based treatment (MBT), she should not attempt to work with Lily now.

3. Disagree, saying that this work is basic and anyone can do it.
4. Disagree, explaining that patients with BPD usually get better and Sarah can likely be very helpful if she follows some key guiding principles and works closely with a supervisor who can help Sarah learn and apply them.

Discussion

Lily's presentation is common both with regard to its symptomatology and (within a mental health system) in its historical details. Patients with BPD are often unaware of their diagnosis and not receiving appropriate care for the disorder. BPD has approximately 15% bidirectional comorbidity with bipolar disorder [1] but is frequently misdiagnosed as bipolar disorder by patients, their families and friends, and even clinicians [2]. This leads to unnecessary or even harmful trials of medication, and discrepant expectations by patients, families, and clinicians about the course and nature of treatment.

While Lily has likely had symptoms consistent with BPD since her teen years, living with BPD into one's 30s without having received the diagnosis is not uncommon. Causes include the issues of misdiagnosis discussed above as well as clinicians' avoidance of giving the diagnosis for a variety of reasons including fear of stigma, concern about making a diagnosis they do not feel equipped to treat, or worries about insurance coverage for BPD treatment. Problematic drinking is often a direct symptom of BPD, but at the same time can mask the diagnosis when patients, families, and treaters ascribe erratic behavior, affective lability, and self-harm to alcohol use and look no further for a comprehensive explanation.

Lilly's experience with cutting is also typical for BPD. First, like most of the maladaptive behaviors in BPD, it occurs primarily in the setting of acute interpersonal stress. Second, while Lily has thoughts of suicide, the cutting was an attempt to find "relief," not to die. Third, her social media posts depicting self-harm illustrate how this behavior often has dual functions of eliciting acute emotional relief and communicating distress to others who might respond in ways that demonstrate care and concern.

Sarah should be told that Lily's case is not hopeless and, at least at this point, does not require specialized treatment or a BPD expert. At least 80% of patients achieve symptomatic remission (no longer meeting DSM-5 criteria) within 10 years [3], and most do so with only informed generalist care. Treatment can improve the chances of, and accelerate, recovery (achieving at least one stable relationship and a stable vocational role). With the proper supervision, a resident can expect change for her patient.

Answers

1. U
2. U
3. U
4. H

Principles and Clinical Pearls

1. BPD is frequently misdiagnosed, often as bipolar disorder.
2. Treating BPD patients is not easy, but usually does not require a BPD expert. In most cases, a dedicated, informed generalist clinician can be very helpful and should expect progress when working with such a patient.

Case Continues...

You encourage Sarah by acknowledging that working with Lily will likely be challenging, but worthwhile, and that improvement is not guaranteed but should be expected if her course is typical of those with BPD. Sarah initiates treatment over the course of several meetings with Lily and begins regular meetings with you to review the case in light of your BPD expertise. She has been able to take a reasonable history.

Lily grew up in a home with a mathematician father who was kind but aloof and awkward. Her mother stayed at home to care for Lily, but suffered from recurrent postpartum depression after Lily's birth and the birth of her two younger brothers. In later years, she took comfort in a daily bottle of wine. Lily felt little emotional support from either of her parents, and felt she had to look out for her brothers.

When Lily was a high-school freshman, her early physical development and natural beauty attracted attention from older boys, and on occasion male teachers. She liked being noticed, but generally felt disappointment in romantic relationships that mostly left her feeling used. Despite this, she pursued many such relationships, often with older men. She began drinking at age 15 to feel closer to her boyfriends. She first cut herself at age 16 after feeling taken advantage of by a teacher. She thought she was in love and wanted to make the relationship public, but he broke things off. She felt abandoned but thought her parents would not believe her or even care about what happened, so found a razor and cut her forearms. Her father was alarmed and brought her to the ED, where she lied and blamed her feelings on a crush on a fictitious boy at school. Her father did ensure that she began seeing a therapist, with whom she did not feel connected.

Lily went off to college and excelled academically in psychology, but continued to struggle with secretive cutting and drinking. After college, she worked in several labs while considering a career in psychology or medicine but she kept getting "thrown off" by men who took advantage of her and left her when she became jealous of their time away from her. Her 20s were thus spent alternating between desperately seeking love and concluding she would never find it. Following a breakup at age 25, she drank for 2 days without sleeping and ended up in the ED agitated and suicidal. She had a brief admission, where she was diagnosed with bipolar disorder, and subsequently had multiple years with various psychiatrists who treated her with lithium, valproate, lamotrigine, and occasional antipsychotics. Little helped, and she kept drinking and acting impulsively. She quit treatment after losing her insurance between job changes. At this point she has been living alone in an apartment funded by money inherited from her grandmother, but has not had a job in 18 months and is no longer thinking about further education.

Sarah feels that she is beginning to create an alliance with Lily but remains concerned about Lily's inconsistent attendance and ongoing drinking. Lily frequently arrives late, sometimes smelling of alcohol. Lily denies she has a drinking problem, though concedes she occasionally drinks to keep her moods even. When Lily recently did not appear for her weekly appointment, Sarah called her at home and heard her slurring her words and repeating herself while claiming she forgot the session and requesting "a phone sessshhhhh…" Sarah initially went along with this request but soon regretted it when the conversation was unproductive and at one point Lily was dozing off. Sarah's supervisor suggested offering more frequent visits upon Lily's request for more time, but Sarah is not sure this would be helpful. Sarah thinks that Lily's BPD is likely driving her drinking but is not sure how to address the issue.

Choice Point 2

In response to Sarah's concerns you:

1. Encourage Sarah to offer more frequent sessions with Lily, to jump-start the therapy and improve the alliance.
2. Advise Sarah to make it clear to Lily that she cannot present to sessions intoxicated, and if she does, the session will be terminated.
3. Tell Sarah that she should decide whether she feels comfortable with offering more sessions.
4. Suggest that Sarah respond as follows: "Before adding sessions, we should examine whether our work is helpful. We need to do this together. We will be able to determine this by looking for improvement in your symptoms, including your cutting and your drinking."

Discussion

Early on in BPD treatments, it is common for patients to wish for more frequent sessions, but not always prudent for clinicians to provide this. The impetus for the wish may be an idealizing alliance or a desire to feel contained. A practical clinical response is to link frequency of sessions to evidence of improvement. This emphasizes that positive change is expected for Lily, and clarifies that treatment should generally only be expanded (or continued) contingent upon it being demonstrably useful. This determination requires ongoing, collaborative assessment by both Sarah and Lily. Treatments that are not working should not be escalated in frequency or complexity, but may need to be reduced or pared down.

Lily's alliance with Sarah already seems to be positive, so Choice 1 is likely unnecessary. Choice 2 sets a helpful limit by pointing out that coming to sessions intoxicated wastes their time and yours. Intoxication directly impairs the very capacities of thoughtfulness, perspective-taking, and impulse control that you are trying to help Lily enhance. Choice 3 acknowledges that Sarah should feel comfortable, but neither guides her in how to determine this, nor encourages her to require Lily to be accountable in determining whether "more is better." Establishing accountability and collaboration around expecting and monitoring change, and making treatment contingent on this change, is nicely communicated in Choice 4.

Answers

1. U
2. H
3. P
4. H

Principles and Clinical Pearls

1. Continuing or expanding treatment should generally be contingent on whether the treatment has proven helpful toward the ultimate goal of "getting a life" outside of the therapy.
2. Assessing progress toward goals is a collaborative activity requiring both therapist and patient input.
3. Learning to identify, reflect upon, and express overwhelming internal experiences is a significant goal of BPD treatment made impossible by intoxication during sessions.

Choice Point 3

How would you advise Sarah regarding Lily's drinking?

1. Make increasing sessions dependent on Lily stopping drinking.
2. Focus on treating Lily's BPD, because her drinking is a BPD-related self-destructive behavior that should resolve once BPD remits.
3. Consider firing Lily as a patient given that her primary problem right now seems to be drinking, not BPD.
4. Require Lily to address her alcohol use with specific treatment (such as a dual-diagnosis partial program) and establish sobriety for 3 months before resuming BPD treatment.
5. Continue to work with Lily so long as she comes sober to all sessions.

Discussion

Comorbidity is extremely common and is one of the great challenges of treating BPD. Substance use should be prioritized as a treatment target when it fits a pattern of dependence characterized by chronic use despite recurrent negative consequences and signs of physical dependence. This occurs in up to 35% of BPD cases, and probably requires substance use disorder treatment and a 3–6 month period of sobriety before BPD treatment can be effective. However, problematic drinking or drug use in the absence of dependence is more helpfully thought of as a self-destructive BPD-related behavior that can often be managed within the scope of targeted BPD treatment.

Choice 2 represents a reasonable stance to have toward Lily's drinking at this time, though it incurs a risk of sidelining a potentially more serious drinking problem she may be minimizing. It thus depends somewhat on Sarah's confidence in her week-to-week assessment of the likely fluctuating scope and harms of Lily's drinking. Choice 4 is reasonable if in fact Lily has a true alcohol use disorder. Though it may be too soon to conclude this, Sarah should be advised to be vigilant to escalating signs and symptoms in this arena.

Choice 1 applies the earlier principle of making treatment intensity contingent on effectiveness to Lily's chief presenting symptom at this time. It would be better on all fronts if Lily stopped drinking, and more sessions could be an incentive in this direction. However, it is unlikely that Lily can suddenly establish and maintain total sobriety, and pledging more sessions only on condition of sobriety runs the risk of conveying an overly simplistic "tit for tat" treatment approach that may fuel resentment in Lily rather than inspiration to change.

Choice 3 is too harsh. Lily's alcohol use is either a dependence that she cannot simply quit in response to Sarah's fiat, a self-destructive symptom of her BPD, or some combination of both. In any of these cases, abruptly firing her does not make sense.

Choice 5 is appropriate at this stage. Alcohol must not be allowed to interfere with therapeutic sessions themselves. If Lily is coming sober to all sessions but her drinking appears to interfere with her overall improvement from BPD, her alcohol misuse will have declared itself as the disorder requiring primary clinical focus (Choice 4).

Answers

1. P
2. P
3. U
4. P
5. H

Principles and Clinical Pearls

1. Substance misuse is common in BPD. Clinicians should respond flexibly, but distinguish whether it represents primarily a self-destructive impulsivity best treated as a BPD symptom or a substance use disorder requiring separate attention.
2. True substance use disorders require specific treatment and a period of sobriety before BPD treatment is likely to be effective.

Case Continues...

Sarah continues to work with Lily after Lily agrees to not allow alcohol to interfere with treatment. However, Lily's drinking continues over the next few months. She ends up in the ED intoxicated and suicidal on multiple occasions, and has two DUIs resulting in the loss of her driver's license. Sarah, remembering your previous consultation, determines that Lily is not improving and that her alcoholism is making effective BPD treatment impossible. Lily reluctantly agrees to attend a dual-diagnosis intensive outpatient program with the goal of achieving 3 months of sobriety and then returning to work with Sarah. She follows through. Sarah is pleased to find that Lily has worked hard on her sobriety, comes diligently to all sessions, and seems more likeable now that she is sober. However, she continues to cut frequently and presents to the ED agitated and aggressive. This is despite Sarah and Lily working collaboratively on a safety plan. Lily insists she becomes immediately overwhelmed, and just cannot use any safety plan other than going to the ED. Sarah, in accordance with her supervisor and your previous consultations, has been connecting Lily's self-harm to interpersonal stressors. These include perceived rejection from sexual partners but increasingly relate to Sarah's vacations. Sarah feels that while it is true that Lily is interpersonally hypersensitive, and Lily is starting to make this connection intellectually, she is unable to do anything differently. Sarah feels the treatment is stymied by Lily's repeated dangerous sexual liaisons, cutting, and trips to the ED. She asks her primary supervisor about how to proceed.

Choice Point 4

Her supervisor should advise Sarah to:

1. Require Lily to get at least a part-time job.
2. Require Lily to join a DBT skills group.
3. Refer Lily to a different therapist.
4. Suggest Lily take the opportunity while she is not drinking to apply to graduate school, because goals are important in the treatment of BPD.

Discussion

Social rehabilitation is an indispensable part of BPD treatment. Improving reflective capacity within psychotherapy may be necessary but is not sufficient for real-world improvement unless patients can then employ this enhanced capacity in a relatively benign community environment that can foster wider cultural learning – such as would be associated with a job or other vocational role [4]. All BPD treatment should assert this principle of requiring steps toward functioning outside of treatment settings, as Choice 1 asserts. Now that alcohol is no longer interfering, it is a reasonable expectation for Lily to begin working and building a life outside of therapy. However, as is depicted in Choice 4, clinicians may overestimate capacities or set goals that are not yet feasible, subjecting patients to painful experiences of failure and contributing to their belief that the true depth of their impairments are not recognized. The end result can be patients acting in ways that seek to ensure such recognition.

Groups are perhaps the most effective and economical intervention in the treatment of BPD. Though widely available, they are often underutilized. DBT skills groups are available and a recent study by Linehan shows that they can be as effective in some cases as the standard full-package DBT [5]. Thus, Choice 2 is an appropriate way to provide Lily additional support and behavioral skills training that could facilitate improved emotion regulation and control of self-harming urges.

While it is reasonable to conclude from Lily's continuing self-destructive behavior and ED visits that the treatment is not optimally working in its current arrangement, there is no reason to conclude that changing therapists make sense (Choice 3). This is especially true as Sarah and Lily appear to have created an alliance that appears both contractual and relational, and there are additional clinical interventions discussed here that Sarah can try.

Answers

1. H
2. H
3. U
4. U

Principles and Clinical Pearls

1. Anchoring the treatment around building a life outside of therapy helps insure that clinical progress will produce the widest possible benefit for the patient's life, social roles, and functioning.
2. Setting goals is important, but should be short-term and feasible to foster a sense of progress and mastery. Identifying longer-term goals may itself be a goal over time.

3. Groups are effective and economical treatments for BPD patients.
4. Change is to be expected. When it is not occurring, the treatment should change.

Case Continues...

Lily reluctantly agrees to joining a DBT skills group. She attends approximately 75% of these groups over the next 6 months, missing some because she is in the ED reporting suicidal ideation (sometimes accompanying "slips" in her alcohol use). She has been trying to work part-time because "Sarah is making me" but has trouble staying employed. Once she walked off because she did not think a customer was respecting her. She also left another job after sleeping with her married boss, and once again felt rejected and used. She can talk with Sarah about the skills that she has been learning in the DBT group but says she is usually not able to use them when distressed. The frequency and dangerousness of her cutting appears to be increasing as Sarah's graduation from residency (and inevitable termination with Lily) approaches. Sarah is discouraged and worried. She feels as though she was not helpful to Lily and is unsure how to help her with the upcoming transition. Traditionally, such cases are passed down from one resident to the next, but she is not sure this is advisable. On the other hand, she does not know what else to do. You agree that the treatment has not been as successful as one would hope, but you remind Sarah that she has done several things that will likely prove helpful to Lily including showing her that she can rely on others, helping her become sober, engaging her in the pursuit of work, and introducing her to DBT.

As Sarah's graduation approaches, you advise that Sarah:

1. Transfer Lily to a new 3rd-year resident so they can learn from Lily.
2. Ask her primary supervisor, who is not a BPD specialist but knows Lily, to take over the treatment.
3. Refer Lily to the residential treatment program within your system that provides a standard DBT package of individual and group therapy plus skills coaching.

Discussion

While it is likely that another resident could learn many of the things that Sarah did from Lily, Sarah's 2 years of work with Lily in a generalist mode (not employing specialized treatments for BPD) appears to have stalled. Lily continues to harm herself and present to the ED with similar frequency, signaling a treatment failure, despite Sarah's commendable efforts. Though many cases achieve remission with generalist treatment alone, at this point Lily has not. Choice 1 ignores this by offering further treatment in the same vein. Choice 2 represents a change in clinician, but Sarah's supervisor is also a generalist untrained in BPD specialty treatments so is unlikely to work in a substantially different model. Choice 3 not only acknowledges that a significant change is indicated, but also acknowledges that Lily is unsurprisingly acutely activated, anxious, and self-injurious in the setting of Sarah's impending departure. Increased structure and containment within a behaviorally oriented residential program is likely to reduce Lily's dangerousness during this time and serves as a sound platform for evaluating next steps in her outpatient treatment.

Answers

1. U
2. P
3. H

Principles and Clinical Pearls

1. Many, but not all, patients improve with a generalist BPD treatment model. Others may benefit from more specialized evidence-based treatments such as DBT.
2. When a patient is acutely activated (angry, anxious, self-injurious), increasing external structure and support by shifting the patient to a higher level of care can be stabilizing.

Case Continues...

Lily agrees on admission to the DBT residential program. At first, she increases her cutting and the frequency of her ED visits, attributing her worsening self-harm and suicidality to Sarah "abandoning" her. Within a month, however, these self-injurious behaviors reduce. She begins effectively using DBT skills coaching from the residential staff to avoid some trips to the ED. On the other hand, she finds her interactions with other patients in the residence a mixed bag. She identifies with them but frequently becomes wrapped up in their conflicts with each other, and with staff. She begins to recognize these peer conflicts and staff departures as "interpersonal stressors" leading to cutting.

The suicide of another resident by self-immolation leads Lily to uncharacteristically agree with residential staff that she is ready for discharge. Staff conclude that Lily is ready to leave because she is somewhat stabilized, and she has been at the residence for 6 months, the average duration of stay before resuming outpatient treatment. Lily later shares that she lobbied not to leave because she was doing better, but "because I was doing worse, and I wanted out. Those bastards let that girl kill herself, so why should I trust them to take care of me?"

As an outpatient once again, Lily continues to seem unable to maintain a steady job, and thinks of it as "pointless, anyway." She continues DBT treatment, but only attends half of her group sessions. Her highly experienced individual therapist still cannot get her to use DBT skills when distressed. She continues to cut and overdose instead of using skills, without calling the designated after-hours skills coaches available to her. She has been hospitalized twice in the course of 6 months since ending residential treatment.

Her therapist seeks you out for consultation and reports Lily is "taking up resources in the DBT clinic but not actually applying DBT." She asks you to consider working with Lily in a different specialized BPD treatment approach in which you are trained, mentalization-based treatment (MBT). She reports Lily had heard some things about MBT from Sarah during their therapy, and is now saying "MBT sounds better for me than all this skills crap." You agree to meet with Lily.

After a few missed appointments, you meet with Lily. She appears older than her 33 years would suggest. You note multiple "goth" tattoos on her arms, some covering deep scars. She has other obvious scars, multiple ear and eyebrow piercings, and an outfit made up of revealing leather shorts, tank top, and fishnet stockings. She recognizes your name from your work with other patients she knows, and from her work with Sarah. She sarcastically states you obviously have everyone fooled. When you ask why, she angrily quips "you were supposed to help Sarah and those others help me, and I'm still a mess." You say, "well, I guess I haven't fooled you." She laughs, and relaxes. You discuss her treatment and why she thinks it is not working. She appreciates that you are "cutting the crap, because no one else will admit this is going nowhere." She proclaims, "I'm too fucked up – I can't be helped, especially by all this wise-mind bullshit. I know all these skills, but I'll never use them because it's insulting." You indicate you are unsure why others trying to help her is insulting, but go on to discuss what she knows about MBT. She has a basic understanding from her own reading and says she likes that "it wouldn't treat me like a child."

You both agree to a trial of MBT, on the premise that generalist BPD treatment and one specialized BPD treatment (DBT) have already been tried and found insufficient. Things start well, with Lily attending both individual and group MBT sessions. She is likeable, intelligent, reflective in individual sessions, and insightful with other group members. Unfortunately, she soon resumes her pattern of deep and dangerous cutting, leading to repeated ED visits. For the most part, she is not hospitalized. However, her repeated presentations over the years are causing increasing consternation throughout the hospital system. ED doctors are frustrated and have scheduled meetings with you and risk management and ethics committees about setting parameters for how they should approach her. An individually tailored plan of care is developed for the ED, but is not always applied consistently.

Lily seems to demonstrate balanced reflection about herself and others in treatment sessions, but not in the face of acute interpersonal stress leading up to bouts of self-harm. She continues to reflexively cut herself to feel better, but recently progressed to swallowing sharp objects after cutting seemed to no longer bring sufficient relief. She got the idea from another patient in the ED. She has needed a number of surgical procedures to retrieve ingested needles and razors. All of this hospital time has kept her from sustaining even part-time work. It is now a year and half into her MBT treatment, and though she seems to intellectually grasp mentalizing, she has not been able to flexibly apply it in a way that helps her life improve. Your MBT team notes she is approaching the completion of standard treatment duration.

Choice Point 5

Your team considers how to proceed, and suggests that you:

1. Make an exception for Lily by prolonging the duration of her time in MBT.
2. Transfer Lily to long-term inpatient or residential treatment in a private-pay facility.
3. Refer Lily to a third form of specialized BPD treatment known as transference-focused psychotherapy (TFP), because its focus on angry affect seems to fit her aggressive presentation and it is a treatment she has not yet tried.
4. Reduce the intensity of services being offered to Lily, as she has reached a point of engaging ineffectively with expensive, scarce BPD treatment resources – with the caveat that you will reevaluate her over time and consider resuming treatment if she demonstrates a greater commitment to using treatment to build a different life for herself.

Discussion

The chronicity and severity of Lily's clinical course is uncommon. A minority of patients with BPD do not remit despite aggressive treatment. MBT is an effective evidence-based treatment, but the evidence is for either day hospital treatment or an 18-month course of outpatient treatment [6–8]. There is no good reason to think that extending Lily's current course of treatment will be helpful for Lily (Choice 1). You also worry that creating exceptions for her could harmfully communicate a comfort with lowering expectations for her. MBT is a limited treatment resource with a wait-list of other patients in your clinic hoping for an opportunity to be enrolled. There are long-term treatment centers advertising treatment for BPD (Choice 2) but have little evidence supporting their effectiveness – especially if those centers do not utilize one of the evidence-based treatments described above. Lily has already had intensive DBT-based residential treatment without much success.

In a head-to-head comparative study, TFP (Choice 3) was approximately as effective as DBT [9], and it is something that Lily has not tried. There is reason to believe that her anger and aggression could be uniquely, and perhaps more effectively, treated by TFP. On the other hand, TFP is not available in or near your clinic, is generally very expensive (two private-pay sessions per week), and Lily's swallowing behaviors might preclude acceptance by clinicians providing this treatment.

Given that Lily has not been able to utilize offered treatments for several years to make lasting change, it does not seem useful for her to continue indefinitely in either of the specialty BPD treatments available in your hospital system. Given the waitlist full of other patients awaiting Lily's slot in the MBT program, it seems prudent to reduce the intensity of her treatment toward the minimal level of involvement necessary for preventing further worsening of her course (Choice 4).

Answers

1. U
2. P
3. P
4. H

Principles and Clinical Pearls

1. Change is expected. When it is not happening, it is appropriate to reexamine the treatment through the lenses of peer supervision and expert consultation.
2. In cases of more chronic and severe BPD, routinely discussing your work with peers, supervisors, and expert consultants is essential to prevent the potentially harmful exceptionalism of offering specialized, resource-intensive treatment indefinitely with low expectation for change.

Case Continues...

After lengthy discussion with your clinical team, your own supervisors, and expert consultants you have a frank discussion with Lily. She agrees things are not improving, and wryly reminds you that she predicted this would be the case. She agrees that continuing MBT does not make sense as she feels she already "knows how to mentalize." You mention some of the private residential programs but express your ambivalence. She states those would be a waste of time, just like "the DBT residential." You mention TFP and give her some reading about it. On her next visit, she admits she is intrigued by it and recalls she studied the importance of "object relations" in her college psychology classes. She looks into this option, but learns that she would have to move to New York or Boston to receive this treatment and probably could not afford it anyway.

You offer instead to continue seeing her on a greatly reduced basis in supportive fashion. She initially regards this as yet another "abandonment" and does not appear for the first two appointments. Eventually she settles into seeing you approximately once a month. Her self-destructive and occasionally truly suicidal behaviors continue, though decrease slowly over the next few years. She finds sporadic part-time work as a dog-walker and house-sitter that is enjoyable but does not provide much social interaction. She talks vaguely about the long-term goal of going back to school, but takes no action steps toward it. Despite her worrisome behavior, you continue to find her likeable and become more accepting of her unusually severe prognosis, knowing that only limited change is likely.

Summary of Clinical Approach

Limited resources require community-based outpatient clinics to effectively prioritize problems in the comorbid BPD patient. This resource utilization imperative flies against a tendency for clinicians to refer BPD patients prematurely to intensive specialized treatments before they have received adequate trials of generalist treatment. Once non-BPD diagnoses are appropriately stabilized, optimizing the intensity of BPD-targeted treatment for each patient becomes paramount, in order to apportion the limited community-based treatment resources to meet the needs of the greatest number of BPD patients over time. Fortunately, most patients improve and even remit with care from attentive generalist clinicians, or even well-supervised trainees, without need for resource-intensive specialist treatments for BPD. Change is expected. But clinicians must insist early and often that the patient continually collaborate with them to evaluate whether progress is being made. Accountability on the part of clinician and patient is required, and change should be measured against the yardstick of "building a life worth living." As long as this is occurring, treatment should continue.

When progress stalls, or never appears, consultation should be obtained to evaluate whether changes are indicated – either by adding other elements (e.g., groups), changing the level of care, changing clinicians, or "stepping up" a patient into a more resource-intensive specialist BPD treatment if available. Specialty treatments typically require intensive team involvement and should thus be reserved for patients who fail to progress with generalist care. The team-based and more highly structured strategies associated with DBT and MBT allow for an even more judicious attention to monitoring progress. In rare cases where these intensive programs fail to engage a patient or help them progress, specialist teams can help step the patient down from a level of treatment intensity that has proven unhelpful, making space for other patients to enter these treatments off a waitlist. Formal stepped-care models described in the literature can allow clinics with limited resources to reserve more intensive treatment for the minority who truly require it [10].

Clinician Experience
For many residents and clinicians-in-training, treating BPD patients can engender fear and loathing. As a residency training director, I find that BPD nevertheless presents a tremendous opportunity for learning to become an agent of meaningful change in the lives of the patients we serve. Longitudinal studies have shown that BPD has a hopeful prognosis and that engaged individual treaters can effect meaningful change in their course. All residents can learn to provide good enough care through accurate diagnosis, psychoeducation, active

collaboration emphasizing patient accountability, focusing on real-world change, and case management.

Learning effective BPD treatment strategies under close supervision helps trainees learn much more than how to treat one particular disorder. BPD treatment requires residents become familiar with following patients across multiple levels of care (outpatient clinics, partial hospital programs, emergency rooms, and residential and inpatient settings) and symptom domains (cognitive, affective, impulse-related, interpersonal, externalizing, and internalizing). The diagnosis affects patients of all races, socioeconomic backgrounds, and genders. High levels of comorbidity dictate that residents become proficient at diagnosing, differentiating, and treating mood disorders, psychotic disorders, anxiety disorders, eating disorders, other personality disorders, and substance use disorders. BPD's refractoriness to pharmacotherapy requires that residents apply humility and symptom-targeted prescribing algorithms when offering a wide variety of different medications. Finally, managing BPD patients provides continuous opportunities for learning and applying different clinical techniques, including supportive, cognitive, behavioral, interpersonal, and psychodynamic therapies in individual and group forums. Supervising residents in treating BPD thus challenges us to eclectically and pragmatically bring all of expertise to bear. In short, to paraphrase Osler: "She who knows BPD knows psychiatry."

References

1. Gunderson JG, Weinberg I, Daversa MT, Kueppenbender KD, Zanarini MC, Shea MT, Skodol AE, Sanislow CA, Yen S, Morey LC, Grilo CM, McGlashan TH, Stout RL, Dyck I. Descriptive and longitudinal observations on the relationship of borderline personality disorder and bipolar disorder. Am J Psychiatry. 2006;163(7):1173–8.
2. Zimmerman M, Ruggero CJ, Chelminski I, Young D. Psychiatric diagnoses in patients previously overdiagnosed with bipolar disorder. J Clin Psychiatry. 2009;71(1):26–31.
3. Zanarini MC, Hörz S, Frankenburg FR, Weingeroff J, Reich DB, Fitzmaurice G. The 10-year course of PTSD in borderline patients and axis II comparison subjects. Acta Psychiatr Scand. 2011;124(5):349–56.
4. Fonagy P, Luyten P, Allison E, Campbell C. What we have changed our minds about: part 2. Borderline personality disorder, epistemic trust and the developmental significance of social communication. Borderline Personality Disorder and Emotion Dysreguation. 2017;4(9).
5. Linehan MM, Korslund KE, Harned MS, Gallop RJ, Lungu A, Neacsiu AD, McDavid J, Comtois KA, Murray-Gregory AM. JAMA Psychiat. 2015;72(5):475–82.
6. Bateman A, Fonagy P. Effectiveness of partial hospitalization in the treatment of borderline personality disorder: a randomized controlled trial. Am J Psychiatr. 1999;156(10):1563–9.
7. Bateman A, Fonagy P. Randomized controlled trial of outpatient mentaliziation-based treatment versus structured clinical management for borderline personality disorder. Am J Psychiatr. 2009;166(12):1355–64.
8. Laurenssen EMP, Luyten P, Kikkert MJ, Westra D, Peen J, Soons MBJ, van Dam AM, van Broehuyzen AJ, Blankers M, Busschbach JJV, Dekker JJM. Day hospital mentalization-based treatment v. specialist treatment as usual in patients with borderline personality disorder: randomized controlled trial. Psychol Med. 2018:1–8. [Epub ahead of print]

9. Clarkin JF, Levy KL, Lensenweger MF, Kernberg OF. Evaluating three treatments for borderline personality disorder: a multiwave study. Am J Psychiatry. 2007;164(6):922–8.
10. Choi-Kain LW, Albert EB, Gunderson JG. Evidence-based treatments for borderline personality disorder: implementation, integration, and stepped care. Harv Rev Psychiatry. 2016;24(5):342–56.

Dr. Price is the director of residency training in the psychiatry department at Maine Medical Center (MMC), and Assistant Professor at Tufts University School of Medicine. He is a graduate of the University of Pennsylvania School of Medicine and completed residency at Massachusetts General and McLean Hospitals. Trained in Good Psychiatric Management, Mentalization-Based Treatment, and Transference-Focused Psychotherapy, he is director of the personality disorders specialty clinic at MMC where he teaches and supervises psychiatry residents working in a version of a stepped-care model for the treatment of Borderline Personality Disorder (BPD).

Index

© Springer International Publishing AG, part of Springer Nature 2018   221
B. Palmer, B. Unruh (eds.), *Borderline Personality Disorder*,
https://doi.org/10.1007/978-3-319-90743-7

Printed in the United States
By Bookmasters